Obstetrics

The guide and the practice

PART I

SHERIF A.M. SHAZLY, M.B.B.cH, M.S.c

First edition 2015

To my kind parents, my brother, my dear wife and lovely son,

I love you Yousef......

CONTENT

CHAPTER 1
ANTENATAL CARE

STATION 1: ANTENATAL PRACTICE

Antenatal care

GENERAL CONCEPTS OF ANTENATAL CARE

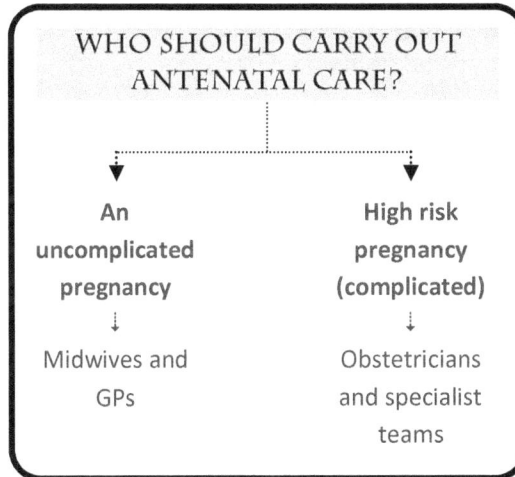

WHO SHOULD CARRY OUT ANTENATAL CARE?

An uncomplicated pregnancy	High risk pregnancy (complicated)
↓	↓
Midwives and GPs	Obstetricians and specialist teams

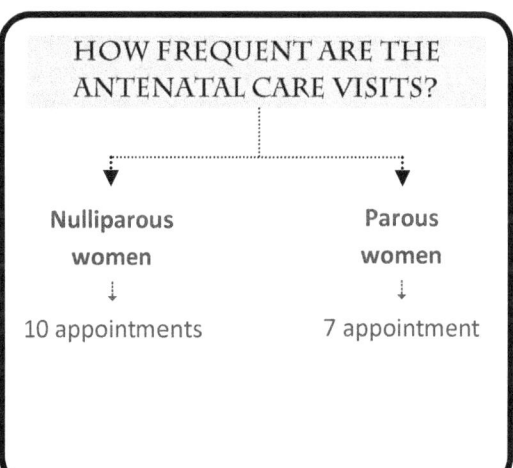

HOW FREQUENT ARE THE ANTENATAL CARE VISITS?

Nulliparous women	Parous women
↓	↓
10 appointments	7 appointment

CONTENTS OF APPOINTMENTS

I. First contact with a healthcare provider

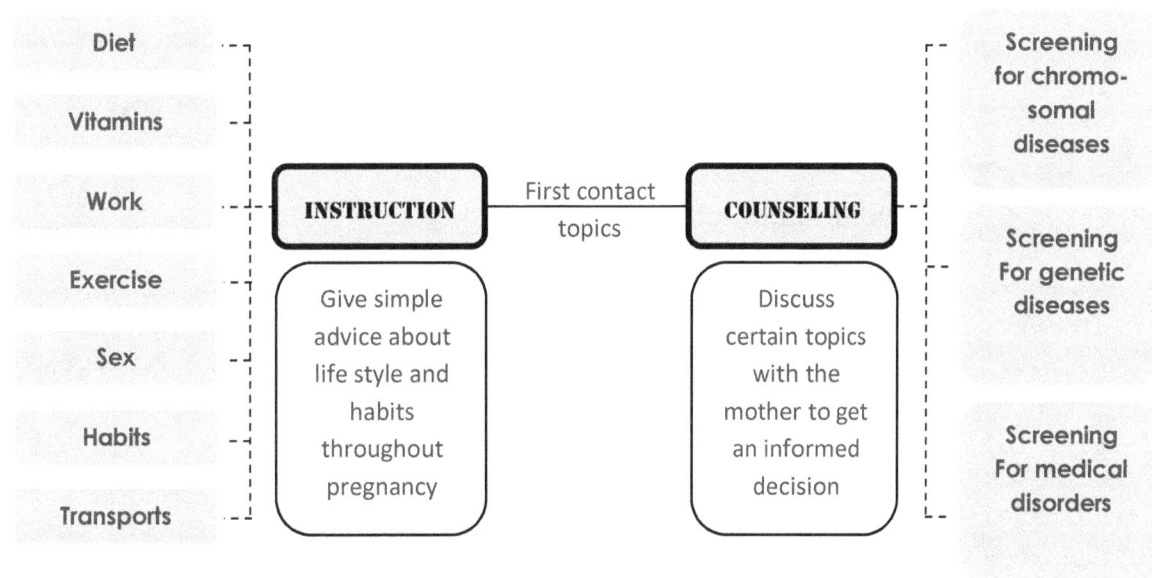

Diet
Vitamins
Work
Exercise
Sex
Habits
Transports

INSTRUCTION — First contact topics — **COUNSELING**

INSTRUCTION: Give simple advice about life style and habits throughout pregnancy

COUNSELING: Discuss certain topics with the mother to get an informed decision

Screening for chromosomal diseases

Screening For genetic diseases

Screening For medical disorders

I. INSTRUCTIONS

Diet
- Follow balanced diet.
- Avoid ripened soft cheese, uncooked or undercooked meals (risk of listeriosis).
- Avoid raw, partially cooked eggs, mayonnaise, undercooked meat (risk of salmonella).
- Avoid liver (high vitamin A).

Vitamins
- Folic acid (400 μg/day) preconceptionally and during the first trimester
- Vitamin D (10 μg/day) during pregnancy and lactation.
- Vitamin A (> 700 μg/day) should be avoided (teratogenic).
- Routine iron therapy is not indicated.

Work
- Reassure that work is generally safe (if there is no specific job risk).

Exercise
- Reassure that moderate exercise is good (based on prepregnancy exercise habits).
- Avoid stressful exercise and scuba diving.

Sex
- Reassure that sex is safe.

Habits
- Give information about smoking risk and support cessation. Nicotine replacement therapy may be considered.
- Advise cessation of alcohol intake particularly in the first trimester. If not possible, it should be at least markedly reduced (e.g. one small glass of wine once or twice weekly).
- Cannabis is to be avoided during pregnancy.

Transports
- Advise that air travel is possible with the following percussions:
  - There should be no medical contraindication e.g. recent sickling crisis.
  - Most airlines do not allow travelling after 36 weeks (33 weeks in dichorionic multiple pregnancy).
  - Compression stockings are effective in reducing the risk of thromboembolism.
  - Vaccinations should be considered if travelling to endemic areas.
- Advise women that the seat belt should be above and below the fetus.

II. COUNSELING

Screening

Offer and discuss screening options (their value, nature, benefits, risks and subsequent management according to the results). The reliability of screening tests should also be discussed. This covers the followings:
- Genetic diseases: (sickle cell diseases and thalassaemias) offered for all women at 10 weeks of pregnancy.
- Chromosomal disorders: (Down syndrome) offered from the 11th week.
- Medical disorders: (diabetes mellitus) depending on maternal risk factors.
- Infections: (Hepatitis B, HIV, rubella and syphilis) at the 10th week of pregnancy.

II. Booking appointment (ideally by 10 weeks)

History

Identify the following problems

| Identify high-risk women through medical, surgical and obstetric history | Identify risk factors for pre-eclampsia and gestational diabetes | Identify past or present severe mental illness or psychiatric treatment | Identify mood and ask about depression (feeling down) in the past month |

Examination

Assessment of the following

| Clinically
Measure height/weight and calculate BMI. Measure blood pressure and test urine for proteinuria | Ultrasound
Offer early ultrasound scan for gestational age assessment using crown rump length (CRL) |

Investigations

Clinical assessment of the following

| Test for blood group | Test for Rhesus (D) status |

Screening

Offer screening for the following

| Hematological screening
For hemoglobin-pathies (sickle cell diseases, thalassaemias) | Infection screening
For hepatitis B, HIV, rubella susceptibility and syphilis. | Urinary screening
For asymptomatic bacteriuria | Chromosomal screening
Offer screening for Down syndrome (combined test) |

Counseling

Offer ultrasound screening for structural anomalies (between 18 weeks and 20 weeks 6 days).

Discussion

Discuss the development of pregnancy
Discuss the plan of care during pregnancy
Discuss proper exercise (including pelvic floor exercise)
Discuss the place of birth and breast feeding

III. At16 weeks

Interview

Discuss the results of screening tests

If the level of hemoglobin is below 11 gm/dl, consider iron therapy

Examination

Assessment of the following

Measure blood pressure

Test urine for proteinuria

Discussion

Discuss the next appointment

Anomaly scan (for structural anomalies): between 18 to 21 weeks

Ultrasound scan for structural anomalies. Fetal echocardiography is considered as a part of the screen

Ultrasound assessment of the position of the placenta should be considered in the same sit

The presence of structural anomaly (confirmed by second opinion) indicates a referral to a fetal medicine specialist.

Some anomalies may not indicate referral (e.g. anencephaly)

The presence of an isolated soft marker is not sufficient to conclude "Down's syndrome".

The presence of an increased nuchal fold (≥ 6 mm) or 2 or more soft markers indicate referral to a fetal medicine specialist.

If the placenta is low lying but minor degree, asymptomatic women should be re-examined on the 36th week of pregnancy to confirm the diagnosis

If the placenta is covering the internal os (major degree), asymptomatic women should be re-examined on the 32nd week of pregnancy to confirm the diagnosis

IV. At 25 weeks – for nulliparous women

Examination

Assessment of the following

| Measure blood pressure | Test urine for proteinuria |

V. At 28 weeks

Examination

Assessment of the following

| Measure the woman's blood pressure | Measure and plot symphysis–fundal height (28th week & on) | Test urine for detection of proteinuria |

Screening

Offer and discuss the following

| Offer re-screening for anaemia (haemoglobin level) | Offer screening for atypical red-cell alloantibodies |

Interference

Offer the following treatment options

| Offer iron therapy for women with haemoglobin level < 11 g/dL | Offer anti-D prophylaxis to rhesus D-negative women |

VI. At 31 weeks – for nulliparous women

Examination

| Measure the woman's blood pressure | Measure and plot symphysis–fundal height | Test urine for detection of proteinuria |

Discussion

Discuss and record the results of screening tests in the previous visit (28 weeks) and offer management accordingly.

VII. At 34 weeks

Examination

Assessment of the following

| Measure the woman's blood pressure | Measure and plot symphysis–fundal height | Test urine for detection of proteinuria |

Discussion

Discuss the past and future

| Discuss and record the results of screening tests of the 28th week | Discuss labour plan, how to recognize active labour and pain management |

Interference

Offer the following treatment options

Offer a second dose of anti-D prophylaxis to rhesus D-negative women

VIII. At 36 weeks

Examination

Assessment of the following

| Measure the blood pressure | Measure and plot symphysis–fundal | Test urine for proteinuria | Check fetal position |

Discussion

Discuss these future issues

| Discuss breast feeding and the good management of breast feeding practice | Discuss the care of the newborn including vitamin K prophylaxis and newborn screening tests | Discuss postnatal care with special concern about the postnatal blues and depression | Offer and counsel for external cephalic version if the fetus is breech |

IX. At 38 weeks and at 40 weeks (for nulliparous women)

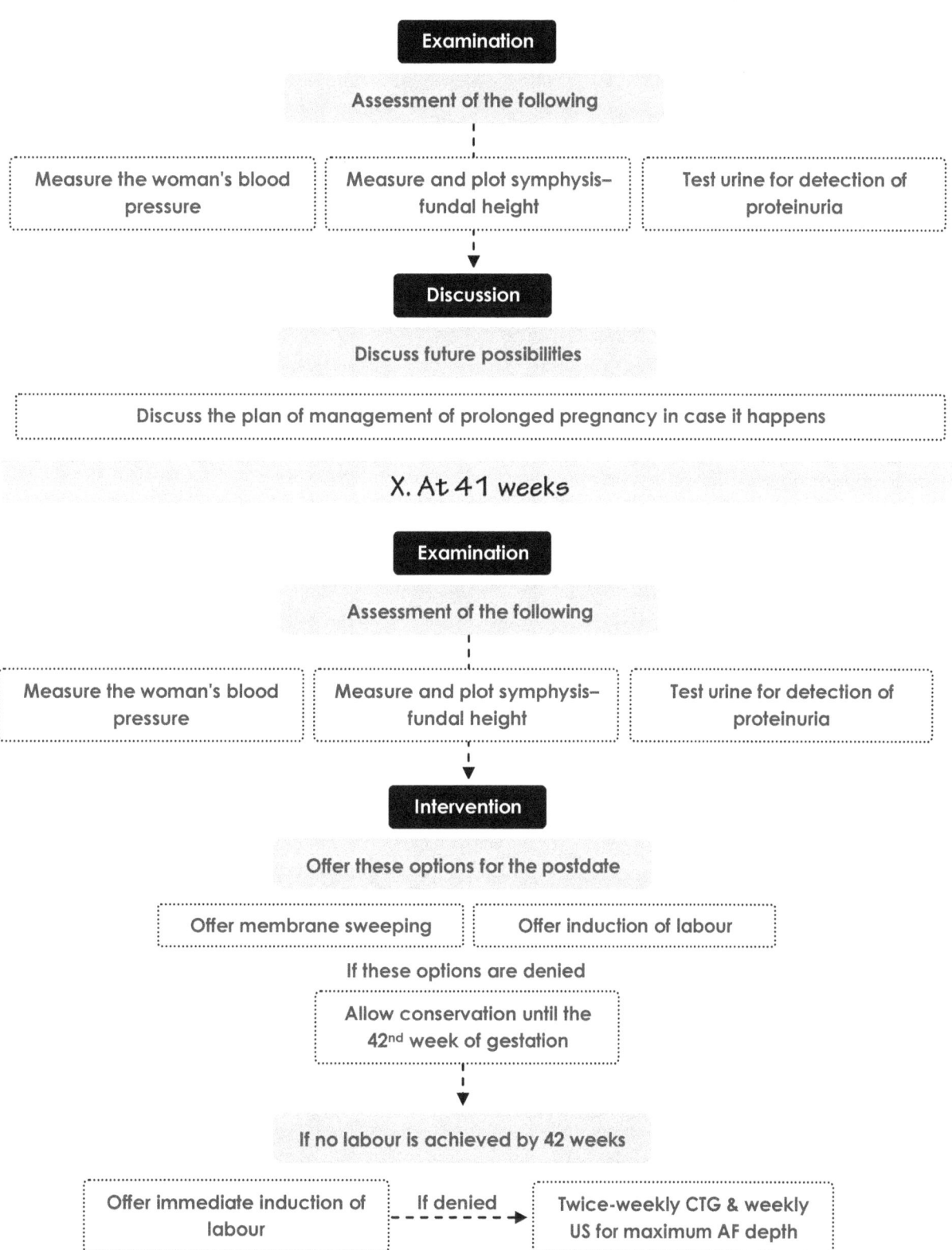

Examination

Assessment of the following

| Measure the woman's blood pressure | Measure and plot symphysis–fundal height | Test urine for detection of proteinuria |

Discussion

Discuss future possibilities

Discuss the plan of management of prolonged pregnancy in case it happens

X. At 41 weeks

Examination

Assessment of the following

| Measure the woman's blood pressure | Measure and plot symphysis–fundal height | Test urine for detection of proteinuria |

Intervention

Offer these options for the postdate

| Offer membrane sweeping | Offer induction of labour |

If these options are denied

Allow conservation until the 42nd week of gestation

If no labour is achieved by 42 weeks

| Offer immediate induction of labour | If denied | Twice-weekly CTG & weekly US for maximum AF depth |

MANAGEMENT OF COMMON SYMPTOMS

Nausea and vomiting

- Reassurance: Most cases of nausea and vomiting resolve spontaneously within 16 to 20 weeks (no poor pregnancy outcome).
- Treatment: If a woman asks for treatment:
  - Non-pharmacologic: ginger - acupressure.
  - Pharmacological: antihistamines.

Constipation

Diet modification including bran or wheat fiber is usually sufficient.

Vaginal discharge

- Reassurance: Women should be informed that an increase in vaginal discharge is normal during pregnancy. It should be investigated only if it is associated with itch, soreness, offensive smell or pain on passing urine.
- For vaginal candidiasis: Topical imidazole is given for 1 week (no oral treatment).

Heart burn

- Advice: regarding lifestyle and diet modification.
- Antacids: may be given if heartburn remains.

Backache

Exercising in water, massage therapy and back care classes

Hemorrhoids

- Advice: concerning diet modification.
- Haemorrhoid creams: are considered if there is no improvement.

Hemorrhoids

- Reassurance: varicose veins are a common symptom of pregnancy that will not cause harm.
- Compression stockings: can improve the symptoms.

MALPRACTICE DURING ANTENATAL CARE

During maternal assessment

- Repeated weighing.
- Undue breast or pelvic examination.
- Routine screening for chlamydia, cytomegalovirus, hepatitis C virus, group B streptococci, toxoplasmosis, bacterial vaginosis.
- Routine screening for preterm labour.
- Gestational diabetes screening using fasting plasma glucose, random blood glucose, glucose challenge test or urinalysis for glucose.
- Routine ultrasound scanning after 24 weeks.

During fetal assessment

- Routine Doppler ultrasound in low-risk pregnancies.
- Ultrasound estimation for suspected large-for-gestational-age fetuses.
- Routine fetal-movement counting.
- Routine auscultation of the fetal heart.
- Routine antenatal electronic cardiotocography.

Appendix - I | **Antenatal care visits' check list**

At 10 weeks

Date: / / .

Clinical
Weight:
Height:
BMI:
Blood pressure:
Proteinuria:

☐ Medical/surgical conditions: ....
☐ Risk of gestational diabetes: ....
☐ Risk of pre-eclampsia: ....
☐ Risk of mood disorders: ....

Screening

☐ Screening for hemoglobinopathies:
☐ Screening for Down syndrome:
☐ Screening for HIV:
☐ Screening for hepatitis B:
☐ Screening for rubella:
☐ Screening for syphilis:
☐ Screening for asymptomatic bacteriuria:

Sonography
CRL:
Viability:

Lab
Blood group:
Rh status:

At 16 weeks

Date: / / .

Report of health problems
_____
_____
_____

Clinical
Blood pressure:
Proteinuria:

Anomaly scan report

At 28 weeks

Date: / / .

Report of health problems
_____
_____
_____

Clinical
Blood pressure:
Proteinuria:
SFH:

Lab
HB level: Alloantibodies:

Anti-D serum:

At 34 weeks

Date: / / .

Report of health problems

_____

_____

_____

☐ Information about labour, labour pain and labour plan given

Clinical

Blood pressure:

Proteinuria:

SFH:

Anti-D serum:

At 36 weeks

Date: / / .

Report of health problems

_____

_____

_____

☐ Information about breast feeding
☐ Information about vitamin K prophylaxis and neonatal screening
☐ Information about postnatal period and postnatal care issues.

Clinical

Blood pressure:

Proteinuria:

SFH:

Fetal position:

External cephalic version

☐ *Succeed* ☐ *Fail* ☐ *Not done*

At 40 weeks

Date: / / .

Report of health problems

_____

_____

_____

☐ Plan for postdate management: ....

Clinical

Blood pressure:

Proteinuria:

SFH:

Appendix - II   **RCOG recommendations for special situations**

Air travel during pregnancy

Health hazards

- Ear troubles especially in the presence of nasal congestion (pregnant women have vasodilation).
- Motion sickness (aggravate morning sickness of pregnancy).
- Lower limb edema/deep venous thrombosis (pregnant women have a hyper-coagulable state).

Contraindications

- Severe anaemia
- Unstable fractures
- Recent haemorrhage
- Upper respiratory and ear infections (e.g. sinusitis)
- Serious respiratory disease
- Recent sickling crisis
- Recent gastrointestinal surgery

Instructions

- Avoid air travel from 37 weeks of gestation (uncomplicated pregnancy) and beyond 34 weeks of gestation (uncomplicated dichorionic pregnancy).
- Take appropriate immunisation according to travelling destination.
- The seat belt is fastened under the abdomen.
- Minimize the risk of DVT by the following:
  - Drink fluids adequately.
  - Minimise caffeine and alcohol intake to avoid dehydration.
  - Walk regularly every 30 minutes particularly if the flight is long (> 4 hours).
  - Use graduated elastic compression stockings (if a journey is > 4 hours long).
  - Low-molecular-weight heparin (LMWH) is considered if there is additional risk of thrombosis (Aspirin has no rule).

Exercise during pregnancy

Risks

- Risk of musculoskeletal injuries (pregnant women have increased joint laxity: avoid contact and weight-bearing sports.
- Risk of hyperthermia in the first trimester (potentially teratogenic): core temperatures should not exceed 39.2° Celsius.

Benefits

- Exercise reduces fatigue, varicosities and swelling of extremities during pregnancy.
- Exercise reduces insomnia, stress, anxiety and depression.
- Exercise improves glycaemic control in women with diabetes mellitus.
- Weight-bearing exercise reduces the length of labour and decreases delivery complications.
- Fetal/neonatal stress is less frequent in exercising women.

Exercise program

Exercise during pregnancy can be adjusted by one of these methods:
- *Based on heart rate:* the maximal heart rate should be 60–70% of preconceptional rate (for sedentary women) and 60–90% (for fit women).
- *Based on age:*
  - If aged <20, the maximum heart rate is 140–155 beats/minute.
  - If aged 20–29, the maximum heart rate is 135–150 beats/minute.
  - If aged 30–39, the maximum heart rate is 130–145 beats/minute.
  - If aged >40, the maximum heart rate is 125–140 beats/minute.
- *Based on the talk test:* the woman should be able to talk comfortably during exercise.
- *Based on Borg's rating of perceived exertion:* it is a self-paced scale of intensity of exertion (6 = no exercise and 20 = maximum exertion). The required range is 12-14.
- *Based on the duration of exercise:* sedentary women should start with 15 minutes of exercise three times per week, increasing gradually to 30 minutes 4 times a week, then daily.

Percussions

- Avoid contact and weight-bearing exercise.
- Maintain adequate hydration and avoid hot, humid environment.
- Avoid hypoglycaemia (adequate caloric intake is essential).
- Avoid supine position during exercise after 16 weeks of gestation.
- Avoid over exercise at high altitudes (> 2500 metres). Four to 5 days allows accommodation.
- Avoid scuba dive (fetal decompression sickness).
- Avoid horseback riding, downhill skiing, ice hockey, gymnastics and cycling during pregnancy (risk of fall and fetal trauma).
- Avoid water temperature above exceed 32° Celsius.

Postpartum exercise

- *Uncomplicated pregnancy and delivery:* walking, pelvic floor exercises and stretching are recommended immediately (mild expercise).
- *Complicated or delivered by Caesarean section:* Gradually resume activity after 6–8 weeks.

Warning signs

- Dyspnea, chest pain or palpitations
- Presyncope or dizziness
- Painful uterine contractions
- Leakage of amniotic fluid or vaginal bleeding
- Abdominal or pelvic pain (back or pubic pain)
- Reduced fetal movement
- Headache
- Muscle weakness
- Calf pain or swelling.

Nutrition during pregnancy

Pre-pregnancy diet

- Diet modification for BMI adjustment in women with abnormal BMI.
- Pre-pregnancy folic acid is recommended (400 micrograms/day).

Placenta

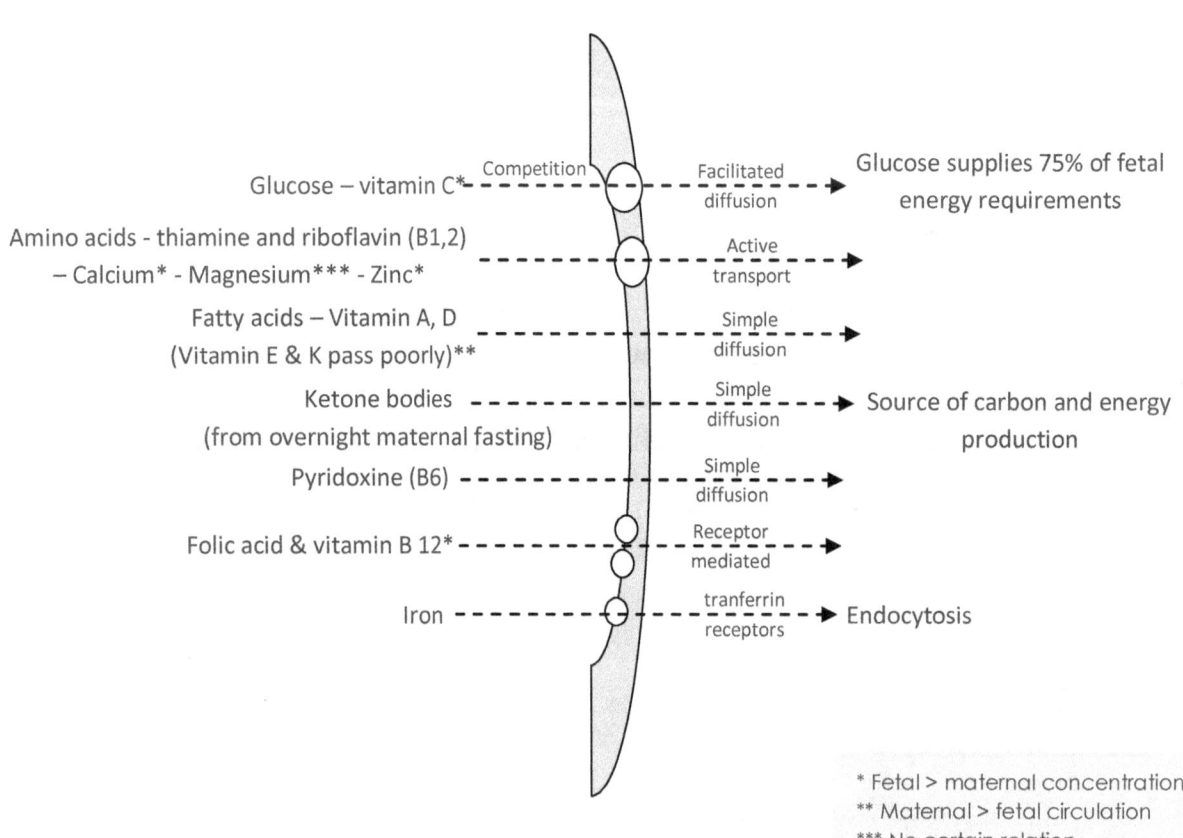

Glucose – vitamin C* — Competition — Facilitated diffusion → Glucose supplies 75% of fetal energy requirements

Amino acids - thiamine and riboflavin (B1,2) – Calcium* - Magnesium*** - Zinc* — Active transport →

Fatty acids – Vitamin A, D (Vitamin E & K pass poorly)** — Simple diffusion →

Ketone bodies (from overnight maternal fasting) — Simple diffusion → Source of carbon and energy production

Pyridoxine (B6) — Simple diffusion →

Folic acid & vitamin B 12* — Receptor mediated →

Iron — tranferrin receptors → Endocytosis

* Fetal > maternal concentration
** Maternal > fetal circulation
*** No certain relation

Pregnancy regimen .... How much to eat?

Pregnant women consume energy variably. The rule is to 'eat to appetite'.

What is needed in diet?

Energy	Protein	Thiamine	Riboflavin
1940 + 200* kcal	45 gm + 6 gm**	0.8 mg + 0.1 mg*	1.1 mg + 0.3 mg**
Niacin	**Vitamin B6**	**Vitamin B12**	**Folate**
13 mg	1.2 mg	1.5 g	200 µg + 100 µg**
Vitamin C	**Vitamin A**	**Vitamin D**	**Calcium**
40 mg + 10 mg**	600 µg + 100 µg**	0 + 10 µg**	700 mg
Phosphorus	**Magnesium**	**Sodium**	**Potassium**
550 mg	270 mg	1600 mg	3500 mg
Chloride	**Iron**	**Zinc**	**Copper**
2500 mg	14.8 mg	7 mg	1.2 mg
	Selenium	**Iodine**	
	60 µg	140 µg	

* (+) in the third trimester only

** (+) during the whole pregnancy

How to supply these needs?

Group I: Bread, cereals & potatoes   **Group II: Fruits and vegetables**   **Group III: Milk & dairy food**

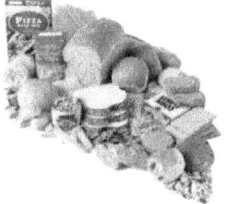   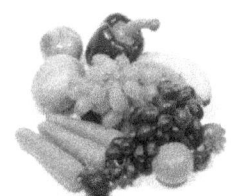   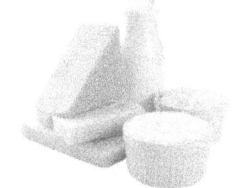

Eat plenty of this group   Eat a variety (at least five portions/day).   Use moderate amounts, low-fat versions

Group IV: Meat, fish & others (beans, eggs)   **Group V: High fat/sugar foods and drinks**

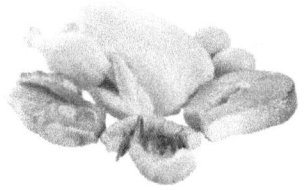   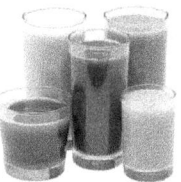

Eat moderate amounts and choose lower fat meat.   Avoid high sugar contents (tooth decay), Eat food with high amount of fat sparingly (use low fat alternatives).

Diet percussions

Liver products

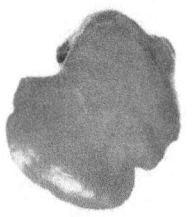

Avoid liver and liver products (excess vitamin A "retinol" which is teratogenic)

Soft cheeses

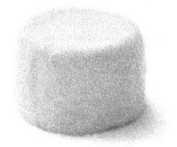

Avoid mould-ripened soft cheeses, unpasteurised milk or pates (risk of listeriosis).

Undercooked meat

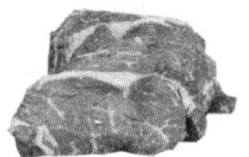

Avoid undercooked meat or salad vegetables contaminated with soil (risk of toxoplasmosis).

Caffeine

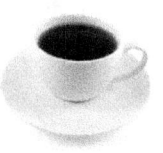

Avoid caffeine consumption > 200 mg/day = 2 mugs of instant coffee (high caffeine is associated with small-for-gestational-age babies and miscarriage).

Oily fish (omega 3 fatty acids)

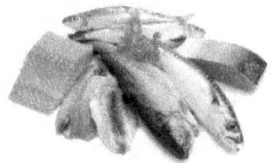

This is controversial (the benefit of omega 3 fatty acids versus the risk of contamination by methyl mercury and polychlorinated biphenyls on the fetus).
Consume two portions of fish a week (one of them should be oily). Limit tuna (four medium-sized cans per week).

Vitamin supplements

Folic acid	Folic acid is given at a dose of 400 micrograms/day before conception and up to 12 weeks of gestation.
Vitamin A	Vitamin A > 700 micrograms should be avoided (teratogenic).
Pyridoxine (vitamin B6)	Not a routine. Vitamin B6 reduces nausea (but not vomiting) in the first trimester and the risk of dental decay.
Other vitamin Bs	Not a routine.
Vitamin C and E	Routine supplementation is not recommended (multivitamin dose is sufficient)
Vitamin D	Vitamin D should be given (10 micrograms/day) particularly in women not exposed to sun adequately, women with BMI > 30 kg/m2 and women who have limited intake of vitamin D.
Vitamin K	Oral vitamin K1 (10 mg daily) is recommended in the last month of pregnancy if there are risk factors for haemorrhagic disease of the newborn

Appendix - III   **Suggested diet regimens during pregnancy**

Breakfast

- 1/2 cup cantaloupe.
- 2 eggs scrambled with 1/4 cup mushrooms with bell pepper and 1 teaspoon canola oil.
- 1 slice of whole wheat toast.
- 1 cup low-fat milk.

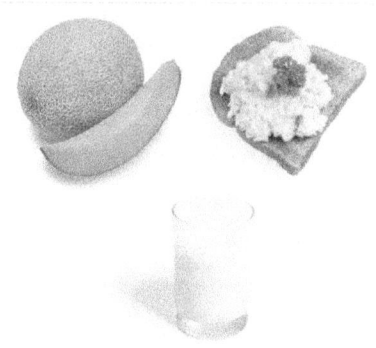

Snack

- 1 large apple.
- 1/4 cup sunflower seeds.

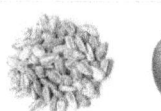

Lunch

- 1 medium baked potato with beans and 2 tablespoons of low-fat cheddar cheese.
- 1 cup of salad.
- 5 whole grain crackers.
- 1 cup of low-fat milk.

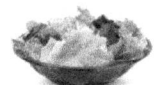 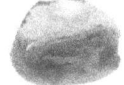  

Snack

- 1/2 cup of baby carrots plus 1 tablespoon of light ranch.
- 3 cups of light popcorn (includes 1 teaspoon oil).

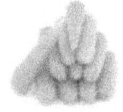 

Dinner

- Half sliced tomato.
- 1/4 sliced avocado.
- 4 ounces grilled salmon.
- 1 cup cooked brown rice.
- 1/2 cup of cooked green beans.
- 1 multi-grain roll.
- 1 orange.

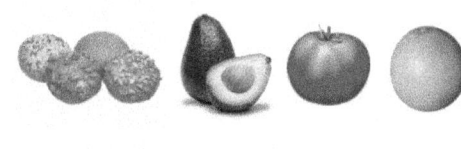 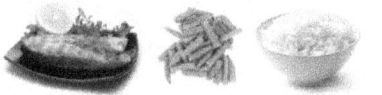

Snack

- 8 ounces low-fat vanilla yogurt.
- 2 gm crackers.

STATION 1: ANTENATAL PRACTICE

Prenatal diagnosis

PRENATAL DIAGNOSIS OF NEURAL-TUBE DEFECTS

Neural-tube defects include anencephaly, spina bifida, cephalocele, and other rare spinal fusion (schisis) abnormalities. However, it is worthy saying that spina bifida occulta (the absence of one or two vertebral arches) is present in 5% of the general population and should not be considered as a risk for NTDs. Approach for prenatal diagnosis should follow these following steps:

Step 1: Whom to assess (the risky zone)

The risk of NTDs is significantly increased in the following situations:
- **An affected sibling:** one to three percent.
- **Affected first cousin (maternal aunt's child):** one percent.
- **Affected first cousin of another type:** 0.3 percent.
- **Mother on valproic acid, carbamazepine and coumadin:** one to two percent.
- **Other risk factors:** include hot tub, sauna, hyperthermia and diabetes.

However, almost 95% of NTDs occur in the absence of recognized risk factor or family history. So, routine screening is indicated in all cases.

Step 2: How to assess (the approach)

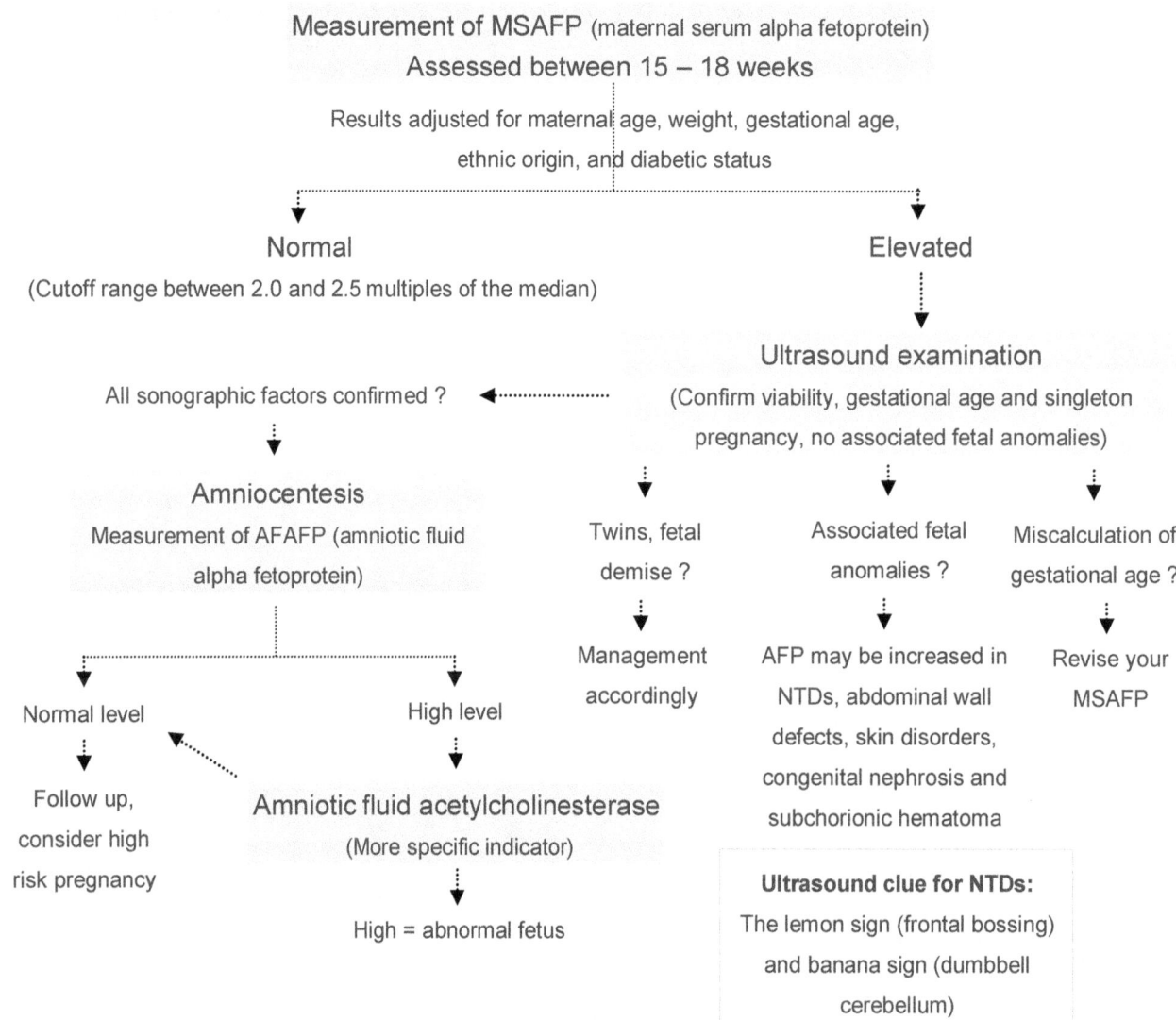

Measurement of MSAFP (maternal serum alpha fetoprotein)
Assessed between 15 – 18 weeks

Results adjusted for maternal age, weight, gestational age, ethnic origin, and diabetic status

Normal
(Cutoff range between 2.0 and 2.5 multiples of the median)

Elevated

Ultrasound examination
(Confirm viability, gestational age and singleton pregnancy, no associated fetal anomalies)

All sonographic factors confirmed ?

Amniocentesis
Measurement of AFAFP (amniotic fluid alpha fetoprotein)

Twins, fetal demise ?

Associated fetal anomalies ?

Miscalculation of gestational age ?

Normal level

High level

Management accordingly

AFP may be increased in NTDs, abdominal wall defects, skin disorders, congenital nephrosis and subchorionic hematoma

Revise your MSAFP

Follow up, consider high risk pregnancy

Amniotic fluid acetylcholinesterase
(More specific indicator)

High = abnormal fetus

Ultrasound clue for NTDs:
The lemon sign (frontal bossing) and banana sign (dumbbell cerebellum)

Fact Box: What should you know before counseling your patient
• The detection rate of NTDs using MSAFP between 15-18 weeks of gestation is 71 to 92%. The false positive rate is 1.2 to 3.9%.
• The detection rate of NTDs using AFAFP between 16 – 18 weeks is almost 99%.
• The lemon sign can also be identified in 1–2 % of normal fetuses.
• Unexplained elevation of MSAFP is associated with an increased risk of fetal growth retardation, oligohydramnios, later fetal demise, and preeclampsia.

Step 3: How to Counsel your patient for further management

Counseling before fetal anomaly screening	All women should be provided with information about the purpose and the possible outcomes of screening and should be allowed to discuss their options, before screening is performed.

Counseling before proceeding to amniocentesis (written consent)	Counseling should cover the following topics:
	• *Name of procedure:* Amniocentesis.
	• *Explanation of the procedure:* The procedure will involve obtaining a sample of amniotic fluid from the pregnancy sac using a needle inserted through the woman's abdomen.
	• *Intended benefits:* Based on this procedure, AFAFP could be carried out. This will increase the detection rate of NTDs to almost 99%.
	• *Serious or frequently occurring risks:*
	  ▪ You should always separate serious from frequently occurring risks for the patient:
	    • *Frequent risks:* mild discomfort at needle insertion site (equivalent to the experience of venepuncture).
	    • *Serious risks:*
	      – Failure to obtain a sample of amniotic fluid (the first attempt success for experienced operators is 94%).
	      – Blood stained samples (0.8% assuming the use of continuous ultrasound guidance and an experienced operator).
	      – Miscarriage (a rate of 1% over the norm is usually quoted).
	      – Fetal injury. It has been described only in case reports. The use of continuous ultrasound guidance may minimize this risk.
	      – Maternal bowel injury. This is also rare.

	– Amniotic fluid leakage: temporary or prolonged. – Chorioamnionitis. Severe sepsis, including maternal death, has been reported but the risk of severe sepsis is likely to be less than 1/1000 procedures. ■ Obese women must be aware that the procedure may be technically difficult and that this could lead to an increased rate of complications.	
Counseling regarding the outcome of pregnancy (morbidity and mortality)	***Anencephaly***	Only 40% stay alive at 24 hours of age, and 5% at 1 week of age.
	Encephalocele	The mortality rate is 60–75% during the first year.
	Open spina bifida	• The outcome depends on: ■ *The level of the lesion:* the higher the lesion, the greater is the neurologic deficit. ■ *Other associated anomalies* e.g. hydrocephalus ■ *Perinatal management* and availability of support services. • If a newborn survives, the major morbidities include developmental delay and the ability to ambulate and maintain continence.
Counseling for pregnancy termination	• All staff involved in the care of a woman facing this decision must be non-directive and supportive. • Even in the presence of fatal fetal condition such as anencephaly, a decision to decline the offer of termination must be fully supported. • Live birth following termination of pregnancy before 21^{+6} weeks is very uncommon. However, women and their partners should be counselled about this possibility. • For a fetal abnormality after 21^{+6} weeks, feticide should be routinely offered: ■ If fetal abnormality is not compatible with survival, termination of pregnancy without prior feticide may be preferred by some women. A fetus born alive with abnormalities incompatible with life should be managed to maintain comfort and dignity. ■ If fetal abnormality is not lethal, failure to perform feticide could result in live birth and survival. The child should receive the best neonatal support and intensive care.	

	• After a termination for fetal abnormality, an organized follow-up care is essential.
Counseling for choosing delivery mode	There is no conclusive evidence regarding the most appropriate route of delivery. However, cesarean delivery is considered for: • Appropriate maternal indications. • Maternal request after counseling. • Hydrocephalus precluding vaginal delivery. • Breech presentation. • Large fetal lesions. For all types of structural anomalies, it was suggested to use the cut off of a lesion measuring 6 cm to decrease the risk of disruption.

PRENATAL DIAGNOSIS OF ANEUPLOIDY

Step 1: Whom to assess (the risky zone)

The risk of Down syndrome is significantly increased in the following situations:
- Advanced maternal age: the cutoff point is set to be 35 years.
- Previous offspring with aneuploidy.
- Parental known chromosomal abnormalities e.g. balanced translocation.

However according to the American College of Obstetricians and Gynecologists (ACOG, 2007), all women, regardless of age, should be offered aneuploidy screening before 20 weeks' gestation.

Step 2: How to assess (the approach)

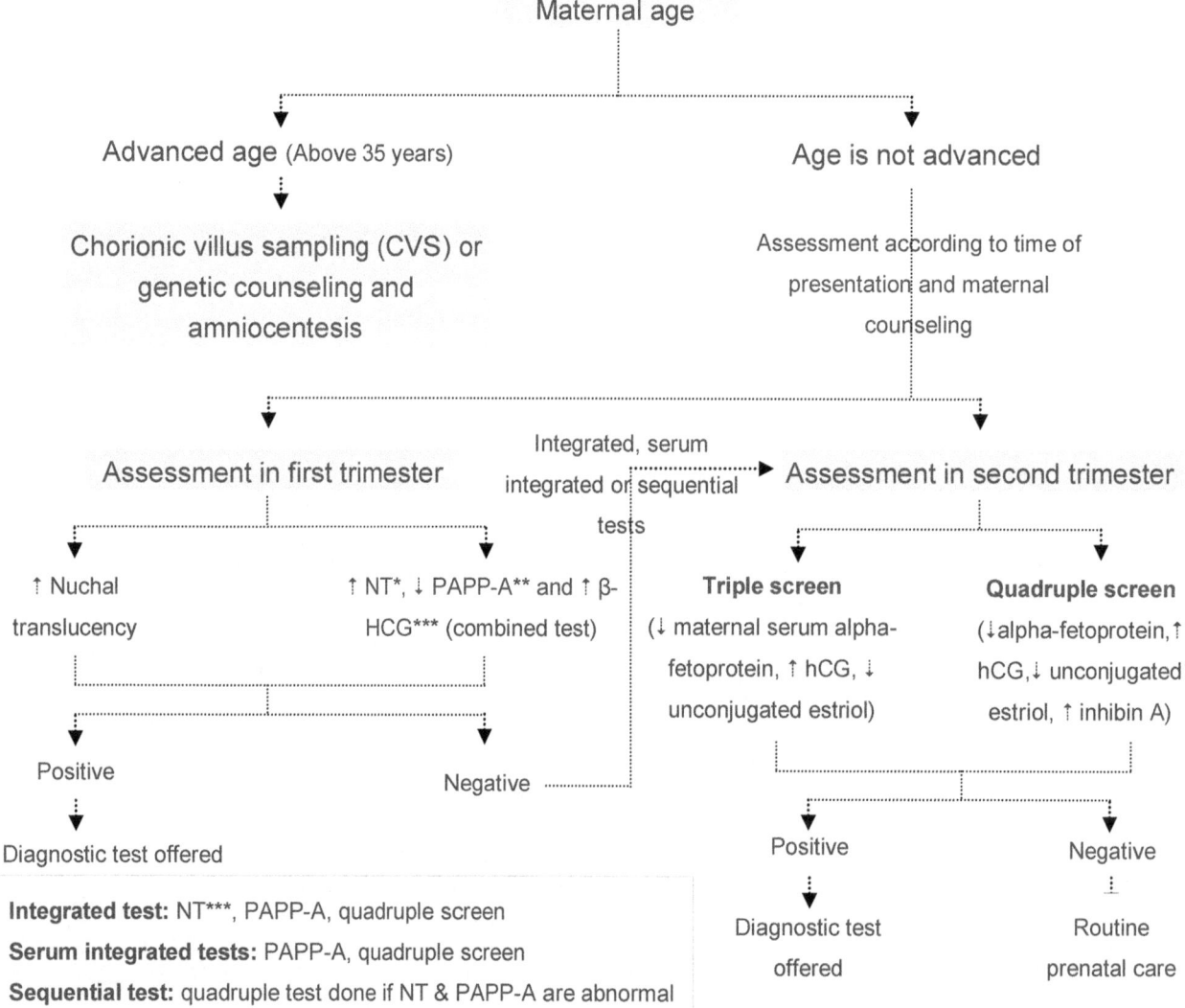

Integrated test: NT***, PAPP-A, quadruple screen
Serum integrated tests: PAPP-A, quadruple screen
Sequential test: quadruple test done if NT & PAPP-A are abnormal

* NT = nuchal translucency; ** PAPP-A = pregnancy-associated plasma protein A; *** hCG = human chorionic gonadotropin

Fact Box: What should you know before counseling your patient

- **First trimester:**
  - The detection rate of NT measurement alone is 64 to 70%.
  - The detection rate of NT measurement, PAPP-A, free or total beta-hCG is 82 to 87%.
- **Second trimester:**
  - The detection rate of Triple screen (maternal serum alpha-fetoprotein, hCG, unconjugated estriol) is 69%.
  - Quadruple screen (maternal serum alpha-fetoprotein, hCG, unconjugated estriol, inhibin A) is 81%.
- **First and second trimesters:**
  - The detection rate of integrated test (NT, PAPP-A, quadruple screen) is 94 to 96%.
  - The detection rate of serum integrated test (PAPP-A, quadruple screen) is 85 to 88%.
  - The detection rate of sequential test is 95%.
- **Second-trimester soft markers associated with Down syndrome:**
  - Nuchal fold thickening
  - Nasal bone absence or hypoplasia
  - Shortened frontal lobe or brachycephaly
  - Short ear length
  - Echogenic intracardiac focus
  - Echogenic bowel
  - Mild renal pelvis dilation
  - Widened iliac angle
  - Widened gap between first and second toes—"sandal gap"
  - Clinodactyly, hypoplastic mid-phalanx of fifth digit
  - Single transverse palmar crease
  - Short femur and humerus

Step 3: How to Counsel your patient for further management

Counseling before Down syndrome screening	Any pregnant woman should be offered screening for Down syndrome. She should be couselled about the tests used and the interpretation of results: • **Blood tests:** have a false-positive rate of 3-5% (you should explain to the mother that three to five children out of 100 who are tested will be diagnosed as having Down's syndrome when they do not). The false-negative rate is 35% (for every 100 cases where a child has Down's syndrome, the diagnosis will be missed in 35 children). • **Nuchal translucency ultrasound scan** has a false-positive rate of 3.5-5%, and a false-negative rate of 30%.

Counseling for amniocentesis and chorionic villous sampling (CVS) - written consent	They should be offered for women aged above 35 years or those with positive screening tests. Choosing one of both procedures depends mainly on the gestational age; CVS is carried out between 11 (11^{+0}) and 13 (13^{+6}) weeks of gestation while amniocentesis is carried out 15 weeks (15^{+0}) onwards. Before proceeding, the following points should be clarified:
	• *Name of procedure:* Amniocentesis or chorionic villous sampling.
	• *Explanation of the procedure:*
	  ▪ Amniocentesis will involve obtaining a sample of amniotic fluid from the pregnancy sac using a needle inserted through the abdomen.
	  ▪ CVS involves aspiration or biopsy of placental villi using either a transabdominal or a transcervical approach.
	• *Intended benefits:*
	  ▪ Chorionic villus sampling (CVS) has a false-positive rate of 1-2%, and a false-negative rate of 2%.
	  ▪ Amniocentesis has a false-positive rate of 0.1-0.6%, and a false-negative rate of 0.6%.
	• *Serious or frequently occurring risks:*
	You should always separate serious from frequently occurring risks:
	  ▪ *Frequent risks:* mild discomfort at needle insertion site (equivalent to the experience of venepuncture).
	  ▪ *Serious risks:*
	    • Women should be informed that the additional risk of miscarriage following amniocentesis is around 1%.
	    • Women should be informed that the additional risk of miscarriage following CVS may be slightly higher than that of amniocentesis carried out after 15 weeks gestation.

Counseling about the risk of recurrence of Down syndrome	Genetic counseling depends on assessment of the underlying nature of chromosomal abnormality, accordingly the risk of recurrence can be evaluated: • For mothers who have had an infant with "classic" Down Syndrome, the generally quoted recurrence risk is 1% (but is higher if maternal age is > 35). • The recurrence risk for mosaic Down Syndrome is 1-2%. • If the child has a translocation, a balanced translocation must be excluded in the parents. However, if translocation is diagnosed, the recurrence risk depends on the type of translocation and the affected partner. • For a balanced Robertsonian translocation, recurrence risk will depend on the affected partner. The recurrence risk if the mother is a carrier is 10-15%, and 2-3% if the father is a carrier. However, In a carrier parent with a 21q21q translocation or isochromosome, the recurrence risk is 100%. • The recurrence risk for de novo translocations is similar to that of the general population but may be slightly higher in some situations; it is estimated to be 2-3%.

PRENATAL DIAGNOSIS OF CYSTIC FIBROSIS

Step 1: Whom to assess (the risky zone)

Despite being more common in certain race groups (non-Hispanic white and Ashkenazi Jewish), the ACOG recommends that CF carrier screening should be offered to all women.

Step 2: How to assess (the approach)

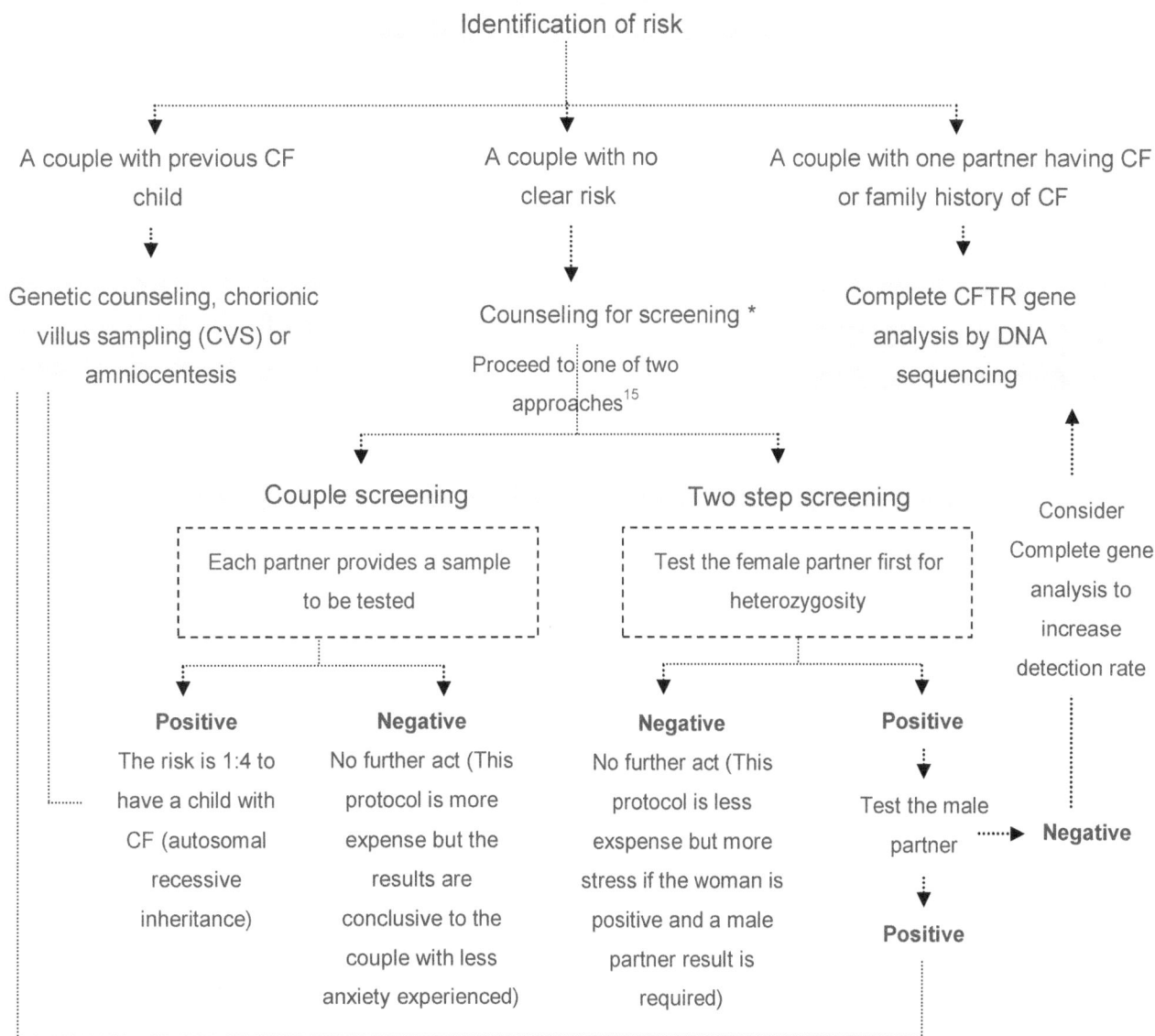

* Screening test is offered using a 23 mutation panel. Complete CFTR is not indicated in classic situations

Step 3: How to Counsel your patient for further management

Counseling before screening	A couple with no risk should couseled for routine antenatal screening of CF. The following information should be offered to the couple: • Cystic fibrosis (CF) is a genetic disorder that causes breathing and digestive problems. Intelligence is not affected. • Cystic fibrosis is an inherited condition that is caused by mutations in the CFTR gene. • Common symptoms include coughing, wheezing, loose stools, abdominal pain, failure to thrive, and, in men, infertility. Treatment involves medication to aid digestion, proper nutrition, and lung therapy. • Individuals with CF have a life expectancy of approximately 37 years. Death is usually due to lung damage. 15% of individuals may have a mild form and live an average of 56 years. • More than 1,700 mutations have been identified in the gene for CF. Screening for the 23 most common mutations is available. The risk of being a carrier depends on an individual's race and ethnicity and family history. Cystic fibrosis is most common in non-Hispanic white individuals and people of Ashkenazi Jewish ancestry.
Counseling for amniocentesis and chorionic villous sampling (CVS) - written consent[8]	See under Down syndrome
Counseling about recurrence risk of cystic fibrosis	You should understand the pattern of inheritance of autosomal recessive diseases to be able to explain the risk of recurrence. Generally, when a woman and her partner are both carriers of a mutation in the CFTR gene, they have a 1 in 4 chance of having a child with CF.

> **PRENATAL DIAGNOSIS OF**
> **HAEMOGLOBINOPATHIES**

Step 1: Whom to assess (the risky zone)

Screening for hemoglobinopathies should be offered to couples with positive family history of patients or carriers with thalassemia. Couples with previous thalaseemia child should be offered genetic counseling. Screening for antenatal thalassaemia is recommended before 18 weeks.

Step 2: How to assess (the approach)

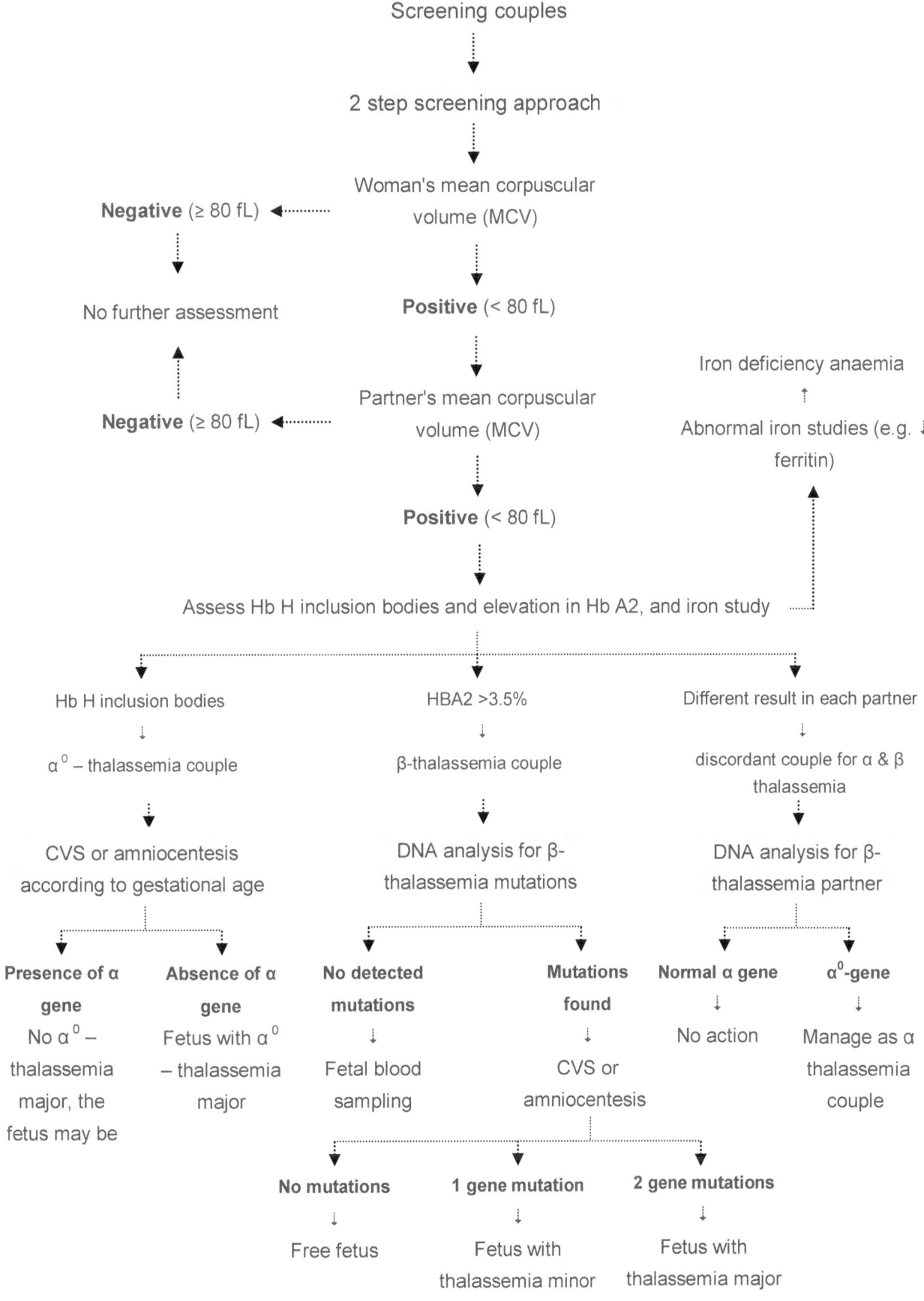

Screening couples

2 step screening approach

Woman's mean corpuscular volume (MCV)

Negative (≥ 80 fL) ◄········

No further assessment

Positive (< 80 fL)

Partner's mean corpuscular volume (MCV)

Iron deficiency anaemia

Abnormal iron studies (e.g. ↓ ferritin)

Negative (≥ 80 fL) ◄·········

Positive (< 80 fL)

Assess Hb H inclusion bodies and elevation in Hb A2, and iron study

Hb H inclusion bodies	HBA2 >3.5%	Different result in each partner
α^0 – thalassemia couple	β-thalassemia couple	discordant couple for α & β thalassemia
CVS or amniocentesis according to gestational age	DNA analysis for β-thalassemia mutations	DNA analysis for β-thalassemia partner

Presence of α gene
No α^0 – thalassemia major, the fetus may be

Absence of α gene
Fetus with α^0 – thalassemia major

No detected mutations
Fetal blood sampling

Mutations found
CVS or amniocentesis

Normal α gene
No action

α^0-gene
Manage as α thalassemia couple

No mutations
Free fetus

1 gene mutation
Fetus with thalassemia minor

2 gene mutations
Fetus with thalassemia major

Step 3: How to Counsel your patient for further management

Counseling during risk assessment	• For couples with low MCV, blood tests cannot confidently exclude that both partners are alpha thalassaemia minor carriers. Further tests are required. • For alpha-beta couples, this means that the couples are carriers of different types of thalassaemias, further tests are required to confidently exclude alpha thalassaemia. • For alpha-alpha couples, alpha-alpha beta couples and low MCV couples, infants with alpha thalassaemia major may die before or shortly after birth. The pregnant women is at risk of serious illness such as high blood pressure and convulsions. • For beta/beta couples, newborns with beta thalassaemia major will gradually develop severe anaemia a few months after birth. They will need life-long blood transfusion and special treatment (iron chelation) to minimize accumulation of iron inside the body, otherwise they will die.
Counseling for CVS and amniocentesis	See under Down syndrome. The tests are 100% definitive in most cases.
Counseling for recurrence risk	If both partners are thalassaemia minor of the same variety, the risk of recurrence is 25% of the offsprings.

CHAPTER 2
FETOLOGY

STATION 2: FETOLOGY

Reduced fetal movement

BACKGROUND   *What obstetrician should basically know about fetal movement*

Definition

Maternal perception of any discrete kick or flutter

Significance

- *Normal perception of fetal movement:* indicates proper function of fetal central nervous and musculoskeletal systems.
- *Abnormal perception of fetal movement:* is a warning sign of fetal death in half cases.

Influencing factors

- **Maternal position:** perception is optimal when lying down, lowest when standing.
- **Placental position:** perception is decreased if the placenta is anterior.
- **Fetal position:** perception is less when fetal back is anterior.
- **Sedating drugs:** reduce maternal perception of fetal movement.
- **Carbon dioxide (smoking):** reduces maternal perception of fetal movement.
- **Antenatal corticosteroids:** temorarly reduce perception of fetal movement.
- **Major malformations:** e.g. *Anencephaly* may increase fetal movement.

Normal pattern

- **Onset:** between 18 and 20 weeks of gestation (16-20 weeks according to partiy).
- **Progress of fetal movement:** frequency increases until the 32nd week then becomes stationary.
- **Frequency of fetal movement:** The average number at term is 31 (16 - 45) per hour.
- **Diurnal Variations:** pereption peaks in the afternoon and evening periods.
- **Fetal sleep cycles:** occur regularly (20–40 minutes for each).

| APPROACH | *How obstetricians should deal with these cases in a stepwise manner* |

Woman with reduced fetal movement

Gestational age < 24 weeks

Recently reduced

Confirm fetal cardiac activity with Doppler device

Never felt

Fetal medicine specialist consultation (neuro-muscular disorders?)

RFM is confirmed by history

1st: exclude IUFD with Doppler

Absent FHS

FHS present

Confirm IUFD by ultrasound

Gestational age > 28 weeks

History

Exclude risk factors of stillbirth and placental insufficiency

Confirm woman's complaint by history

RFM is uncertain by history

- Advise her to lie on the left side and focus for 2 hours.
- If she does not feel 10 or more discrete movements, she should contact maternity unit at once.

Cardiotocograph to exclude fetal compromise

Normal

Suspicious/pathological

Management according to local protocols

Gestational age 24-28 weeks

1st: confirm fetal cardiac activity with Doppler

2nd: history taking (exclude risk factors for stillbirth or placental insufficiency)

3rd: examination (fundal level and symphysis fundal height)

4th: Ultrasound assessment of examination is suspicious of FGR

RFM is excluded by history

- Offer FHS auscultation
- Reassure/perform a routine antenatal assessment

| No risk factor or suspicion of FGR or stillbirth / fetal movement resolved | **History & exam** | Risk factor or suspicion of FGR or stillbirth / RFM persists |

- Reassurance.
- An advice about future episodes: If she cannot account 10 movements in 2 hours, she should contact maternity unit.

Ultrasound assessment of abdominal circumference, estimated fetal weight and amniotic fluid volume

Normal

Abnormality in the scan

History

- **Analysis and confirmation of RFM:**
  - Is it reduced or absent?
  - The duration: for how long RFM is observed?
  - Is it the first occasion or recurrent?
- **Risk factors of stillbirth:**
  - Extremes of maternal age.
  - Primiparity.
  - Racial/ethnic factors.
  - Obesity and smoking.
  - Known FGR, hypertension, diabetes, placental insufficiency.
  - Recurrent RFM.
  - Congenital malformation.
  - Poor obstetric history (e.g.FGR and stillbirth).
  - Genetic factors.
- **Risk factors of FGR.**

Examination

- **Assessment of blood pressure (and proteinuria):** Pre-eclampsia is associated with placental dysfunction.
- **Auscultation of fetal heart:**
  - Auscultation of the fetal heart using a handheld Doppler device is made to exclude fetal death.
  - The fetal heart beat is differentiated from the maternal heart beat by the following:
    - The difference between the fetal heart rate and the maternal pulse rate.
    - Ultrasound assessment of fetal cardiac activity in case of doubt.
- **Assessment of fetal size (SGA):**
  Clinical detection of SGA fetuses is done by:
  - Abdominal palpation.
  - Measurement of symphysis–fundal height (customized fundal height chart is recommended by RCOG).
  - Ultrasound biometry (particularly when clinical examination is difficult e.g. increased body mass index.

Investigations

- **Cardiotocograph (CTG):**
  - *Indication:* when history confirms RFM after 28 weeks and Doppler device confirms fetal viability.
  - *The procedure:* CTG monitoring is made initially for at least 20 minutes, computer systems for interpretation of CTG are more accurate than clinical experts.
  - *Normal findings:* The presence of a normal fetal heart rate pattern (fetal heart rate accelerations coinciding with fetal movements) indicates a healthy fetus.
  - *Abnormalities:* No acceleration for more than 80 minutes suggests fetal compromise.

Investigations (cont.)

- **Ultrasound scanning:**
  - *Indication:* Ultrasound scan assessment in indicated in women with RFM after 28 weeks of gestation if:
    - ◆ RFM persists despite a normal CTG or
    - ◆ Any additional risk factors for FGR/stillbirth.
  - *Timing:* If indicated, it should be performed within 24 hours of initial assessment.
  - *Procedure:*
    - ◆ Assessment of abdominal circumference and/or estimated fetal weight to detect the SGA fetus.
    - ◆ Assessment of amniotic fluid volume.
    - ◆ Assessment of fetal morphology (if not previously performed). This should be accepted by the woman.
  - ***Combined CTG and ultrasound:*** are recommended within 2 hours (if women reported no fetal movements) and within 12 hours (if they reported RFM).
- **The biophysical profile (BPP):** the rule of BPP in these cases is controversial.

Fact Box

- Formal fetal movement counting should not be recommended routinely because:
  - There is wide range of normal fetal count.
  - Warning limits are based mainly on high-risk pregnancy studies and not on normal pregnancy.
- Women with recurrent RFM episodes (2 or more) are at increased risk of a poor perinatal outcome (stillbirth, FGR or preterm birth). Ultrasound assessment is essential for evaluation of these cases.

STATION 2: FETOLOGY

Small-for-gestational-age fetus

| **BACKGROUND** | *What obstetrician should basically know about SGA fetus* |

Definition

SGA fetus is a fetus that does not reach a specific biometry or estimated weight by a specific gestational age. This fetus lies below the 10th centile for abdominal circumference and estimated birth weight for the gestational age.

Causes

- **Fetal growth restriction (FGR):** 30-50%
- **Fetuses that are constitutionally small:** 50 – 70%.

The lower the centile, the greater the possibility of FGR.

SGA and FGR

Certain parameters helpt to identify whether SGA fetus is constitutionally small fetus or growth restricted:

- **Ultrasonographic biometric test:** serial measurements rather than single scan can detect the growth and not the size of the fetus.
- **Composite abnormal ultrasound findings:** a small fetus reduced liquor or abnormal arterial Doppler usually indicate pathology.
- **Biophysical tests:** abnormal biophysical tests usually indicates FGR.

APPROACH　*How obstetricians should deal with these cases in a stepwise manner*

Woman with suspected SGA fetus

History

- Gestational age should be confirmed.
- Risk factors for FGR should be excluded

Examination

- Fundal level
- Symphysis fundal height

Serial ultrasound

Identification of uterine size by:
- Abdominal circumference & estimated fetal weight
- Head to abdominal circumference (HC/AC) and femoral length to abdominal circumference (FL/AC) ratios: but they are less important

If abnormal ($< 5^{th}$ centile) → Ultrasound scan for structural defects

IF

Structural defects
Normal liquor
Normal Doppler

Offer karyotyping

If abnormal ($< 10^{th}$ centile)

Umbilical artery Doppler

End-diastolic flow present

Mostly a small healthy fetus
Conservative management as an outpatient is safe. Follow up with twice-weekly CTG and with Doppler not more than one every fortnight.

Termination at 37 weeks (at least)

Absent or reversed EDF

Gestational age < 34 weeks

Gestational age > 34 weeks

Biophysical profile, venous Doppler

Immediate termination (mostly by Cesarean section)

Normal

Abnormal

Daily CTG/BPP and/or venous Doppler

IF

CTG becomes pathological (decelerations with reduced variability).
BPP becomes abnormal (≤ 4).
Abnormal venous Doppler *.

---

* Reversal of Doppler velocities in ductus venosus during atrial contraction or umbilical vein pulsations.

History

- **Gestational age:** diagnosis should be based on reliable gestational age estimation
  - *Sure reliable dates:* the first day of last menstrual period is well remembered, regular cycles and no lactation or contraception are reported in the last 3 months preceding the last cycle.
  - *Early ultrasound scan:* based on CRL measurement confirms the dates.
- **Risk factors for FGR:**
  - *Chronic maternal disease:* e.g. chronic hypertension, cyanotic heart disease, long standing diabetes, smoking and malnutrition.
  - *Inadequate weight gain:* or constitutionally small fetus.
  - *Fetal infection:* e.g. TORCH.
  - *Teratogen exposure:* e.g. anticonvulsants, illicit drugs.

Examination

- **Abdominal palpation:** the step is necessary but poorly accurate.
- **Symphysis fundal height:** It also has limited accuracy, but serial measurements increase accuracy. Customised fundal height chart (by height, weight, parity and ethnic group) can also increase the accuracy.

Ultrasound

- **Abdominal circumference (AC) and estimated fetal weight (EFW):** Below tenth centile threshold for both EFW and AC are the most accurate to diagnose SGA.
  - *Serial measurements:* more predictive than a single measurement.
  - *Customized growth chart:* it has higher accuracy.
- **Amniotic fluid volume (AFV):**
  - *Abnormal values:* AFI (≤ 5 cm) or pocket depth (< 2 cm).
  - *Prognostic value:* AFV has minimal value in diagnosing FGR, but is predictive of increased perinatal mortality if reduced.
- **Doppler studies:**
  - *Uterine artery Doppler:* has limited use in predicting FGR.
  - *Umbilical artery Doppler:*
    - *Value:* it is the primary surveillance for SGA fetuses. It reduces perinatal morbidity and mortality. It should be applied to higher risk population only.
    - *Predictive indices:* The resistance index is the most predictive.
    - *Follow up frequency:* not more than once every fortnight.

Chromosomal analysis

- **Indications:**
  - An AC and EFW < the 5th centile
  This indicates ultrasound screening for structural anomalies. The presence of the following in ultrasound scan may support the possibility of chromosomal defects:
  - Structural abnormalities.
  - A normal liquor volume or a normal uterine or umbilical artery Doppler.
  In these cases, karyotyping should be offered.

Biophysical profile

- BPP is not recommended as a routine. It is indicated only if Doppler findings are abnormal.
- Cardiotocography is not associated with better perinatal outcome.

DELIVERY

How obstetricians should deal with the labor and delivery

Time of delivery

- **When end diastolic flow is present (PED):** at least 37 weeks.
- **When end diastolic flow is absent or reversed:**
  - *Pregnancy exceeds 34 weeks:* deliver immediately
  - *If pregnancy does not exceed 34 weeks:* consider termination of pregnancy if venous Doppler/biophysical profile is abnormal or CTG is pathological.

Route of delivery

Vaginal delivery is not contraindicated in these cases. However, termination is mostly by Cesarean section because these fetuses usually cannot withstand the stress of labour (poor placental reserve).

Instruction of delivery

- Antenatal steroids are given to reduce the risk of respiratory distress syndrome if gestation is below 36 weeks.
- Continous intrapartum CTG monitoring is recommended to reduce perinatal death.

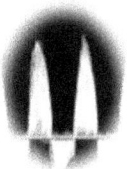

Abnormal arterial Doppler

Average interval (1-26 days)

Interval depends on | *Gestational age*
Hypertension
Abnormal venous Doppler

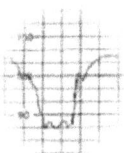

Abnormal CTG or BPP

Fact Box: Ultrasound formula for estimation of fetal weight

- **Shepard's formula:** based on BPD (biparietal diameter) and AC (abdominal circumference).
- **Aoki's formula:** BPD, FAA (fetal abdominal area) and FL (femoral length)
  These are the best formulae (valid between 2080-4430g).
- **Hadlock's formula:** based on BPD, HC, AC and FL (appropriate when the fetus is very small).

STATION 2: FETOLOGY

Intra-uterine fetal death

BACKGROUND   *What obstetrician should basically know about intrauterine fetal death*

Definition
- **Intrauterine fetal death:** no signs of life in utero.
- **Stillbirth:** no signs of life at delivery (died after 24 completed weeks of pregnancy).

Causes

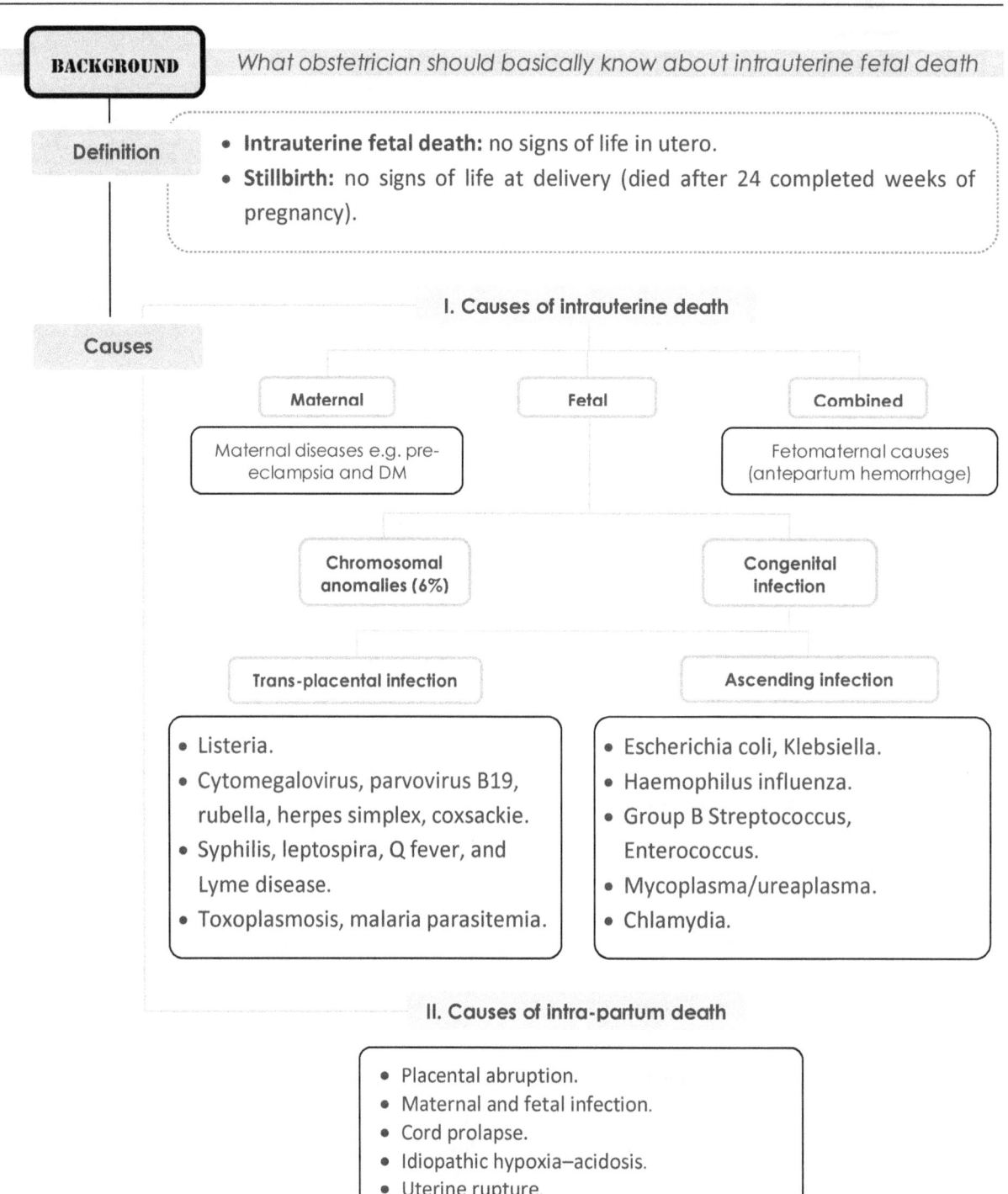

I. Causes of intrauterine death

Maternal — Maternal diseases e.g. pre-eclampsia and DM

Fetal

Combined — Fetomaternal causes (antepartum hemorrhage)

Chromosomal anomalies (6%)

Congenital infection

Trans-placental infection
- Listeria.
- Cytomegalovirus, parvovirus B19, rubella, herpes simplex, coxsackie.
- Syphilis, leptospira, Q fever, and Lyme disease.
- Toxoplasmosis, malaria parasitemia.

Ascending infection
- Escherichia coli, Klebsiella.
- Haemophilus influenza.
- Group B Streptococcus, Enterococcus.
- Mycoplasma/ureaplasma.
- Chlamydia.

II. Causes of intra-partum death
- Placental abruption.
- Maternal and fetal infection.
- Cord prolapse.
- Idiopathic hypoxia–acidosis.
- Uterine rupture.

APPROACH   *How obstetricians should deal with these cases in a stepwise manner*

Step 1	Confirming the diagnosis of IUFD

Suspected IUFD

Auscultation

False positive outcome
30% of fetuses with inaudible fetal heart sound are not finally diagnosed with IUFD.

Auscultation is not conclusive. It should be used to confirm the diagnosis because it carries a high possibility of false results (the same is applied to CTG)

False negative outcome
Maternal pelvic blood flow may give false impression of a viable fetus.

Real time ultrasound

Primary findings
- Absence of fetal cardiac activity (colour Doppler of fetal heart and umbilical artery confirms the diagnosis in case of doubt)
- Evidence of occult placental abruption (only 15% of cases are diagnosed)

Secondary findings
- Collapse of the fetal skull and overlapping bones.
- Hydrops.
- Intrafetal gas within the heart, blood vessels and joints.
- Maceration s and unrecognisable fetal mass.

Diagnosis confirmed

Clinical exclusion of serious conditions

- pre-eclampsia,
- chorioamnionitis
- Placental abruption

Coagulation profile

- Clotting studies.
- Platelet count
- Fibrinogen level

Kleihauer test

The test is to detect large feto–maternal haemorrhage in Rh-negative women

Woman's approach

- Offer to call woman's companion (partner, relatives or friends).
- Discuss the matter with the mother/parents and (accompanied by written information) and support their choice.
- Prepare the woman for the possibility of passive fetal movement (a repeat scan may be offered).

Coagulation profile

- **Rationale:**
  The risk of DIC after IUFD is 10% within 4 weeks and up to 30% after 4 weeks. The risk is higher with maternal sepsis, placental abruption and pre-eclampsia (cause of IUFD).
- **Frequency:**
  Tests are repeated twice weekly if the patient is managed expectantly.

Kleihauer test

- **Rationale:**
  It is used to identify large feto–maternal haemorrhage (FMH) either as a cause or as a result of IUFD.
- **The immunization approach:**

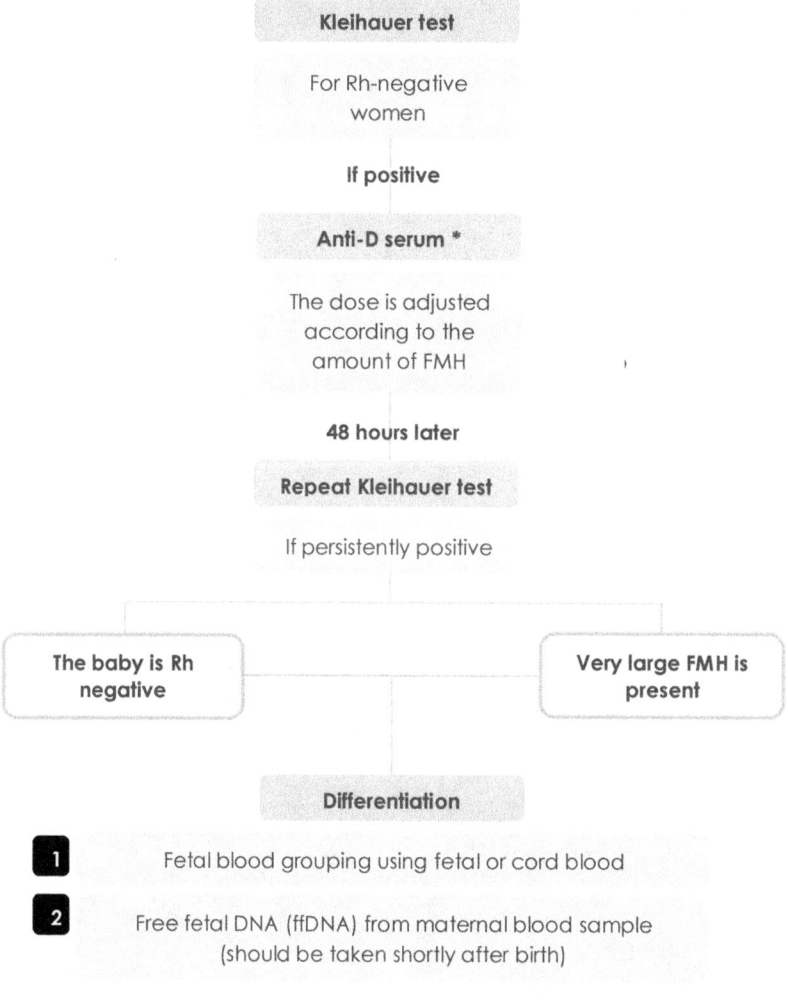

* Anti-D serum should be given within 72 hours of feto-maternal hemorrhage. However, it is still of some value up to 10 days of the accident. It should be considered that FMH may have occurred days before the diagnosis of IUFD.

Step 2   Investigating the cause of IUFD

I   Maternal investigations

Standard laboratory tests

- **Hematology:** platelet count is particularly important in pre-eclampsia and DIC.
- **Chemistry:** it identifies end organ failure in women suffering from sepsis or hemorrhage.
- **Bile salt:** for diagnosis of obstetric cholestasis.

Kleihauer test

- **Rationale:** diagnosis of large fetomaternal hemorrhage as a cause of IUFD.
- **Timing:** it should be before birth before fetal RBCs are cleared from the circulation.

Maternal bacteriology

- **Indications:**
  Indicated only if there is suspicion of chorioamnionitis including:
  - Maternal fever and flu-like symptoms.
  - Purulent offensive vaginal discharge.
  - Prolonged rupture of membranes before IUFD.
- **The tests:** Blood culture, midstream urine, cervico-vaginal swab.

Maternal serology

- **Indications:**
  Indicated for the diagnosis of occult maternal–fetal infection:
  - *Routinely for all women:* Parvovirus B19 (hydrops in not neccessary), CMV, herpes simplex and Toxoplasma gondii.
  - *For women who are non-immune at booking:* screening for rubella.
  - *For women who are investigated for syphilis at booking:* Treponemal serology.
  - *For women who travelled to endemic areas e.g. Africa:* Malaria.

Maternal endocrinology

- **Diabetes mellitus:**
  - *Maternal random blood glucose:* for diagnosis of occult diabetes mellitus (gestational diabetes can be missed because blood glucose returns to normal few hours after IUFD).
  - *Maternal HbA1c:* for diagnosis of gestational diabetes mellitus (gestational diabetes can be also missed because most women have normal HbA1c).
- **Thyroid disease:**
  TSH, FT4 and FT3 are assessed for diagnosis of occult maternal thyroid disease.

Maternal thrombophilia

- **Indications:**
  Indicated if there is evidence of fetal growth restriction or placental disease. However, the association is weak and further considerations in next pregnancy are still doubtful.
- **Protocol:**
  If the tests are positive, it should be repeated after 6 weeks.

Maternal immunology

Test	Indication	Conclusion
Anti-red cell antibody serology	If there is evidence of fetal hydrops	Diagnosis of immune haemolytic disease
Maternal anti-Ro and anti-La antibodies	If there is evidence of hydrops, endomyocardial fibro-elastosis or AV node calcification (postmortem examination).	Diagnosis of occult maternal autoimmune disease
Maternal alloimmune antiplatelet antibodies	If fetal intracranial haemorrhage (postmortem examination).	Diagnosis of alloimmune thrombocytopenia

Maternal urine (metabolites)

Maternal urine is examined for cocaine metabolites (after consent) if there is suggestive data of occult drug use.

II   **Parental investigations**

Parental karyotyping

- Indications:
  - *If postmortem examination:* reveals fetal abnormality.
  - *If fetal genetic testing:* reveals fetal unbalanced translocation or aneuploidy e.g. 45X (Turner syndrome).
  - *If history is suggestive of aneuploidy (no or failed genetic testing):* e.g. previous unexplained IUFD, recurrent miscarriage.
- **Conclusion:** Diagnosis of parental balanced translocation and parental mosaicism.

III   **Fetal/placental investigations**

Fetal and placental microbiology

- Under clean conditions, cord or better cardiac blood (consent required) is obtained. Lithium heparin is added.
- This test is more informative than maternal serology in the diagnosis of viral infections.

Fetal and placental Karyotyping

Karyotyping helps to diagnose aneuploidy and single gene disorders. This helps in:
- Identification of the cause of IUFD.
- Testing in future pregnancies because some anomalies are possibly recurrent.

This can be achieved by: Tissue culture or QF-PCR

Postmortem

Parents should be offered postmortem examination to possibly identify the cause of an IUFD but they should never be persuaded.

DELIVERY   *How obstetricians should deal with delivery of IUFD fetus*

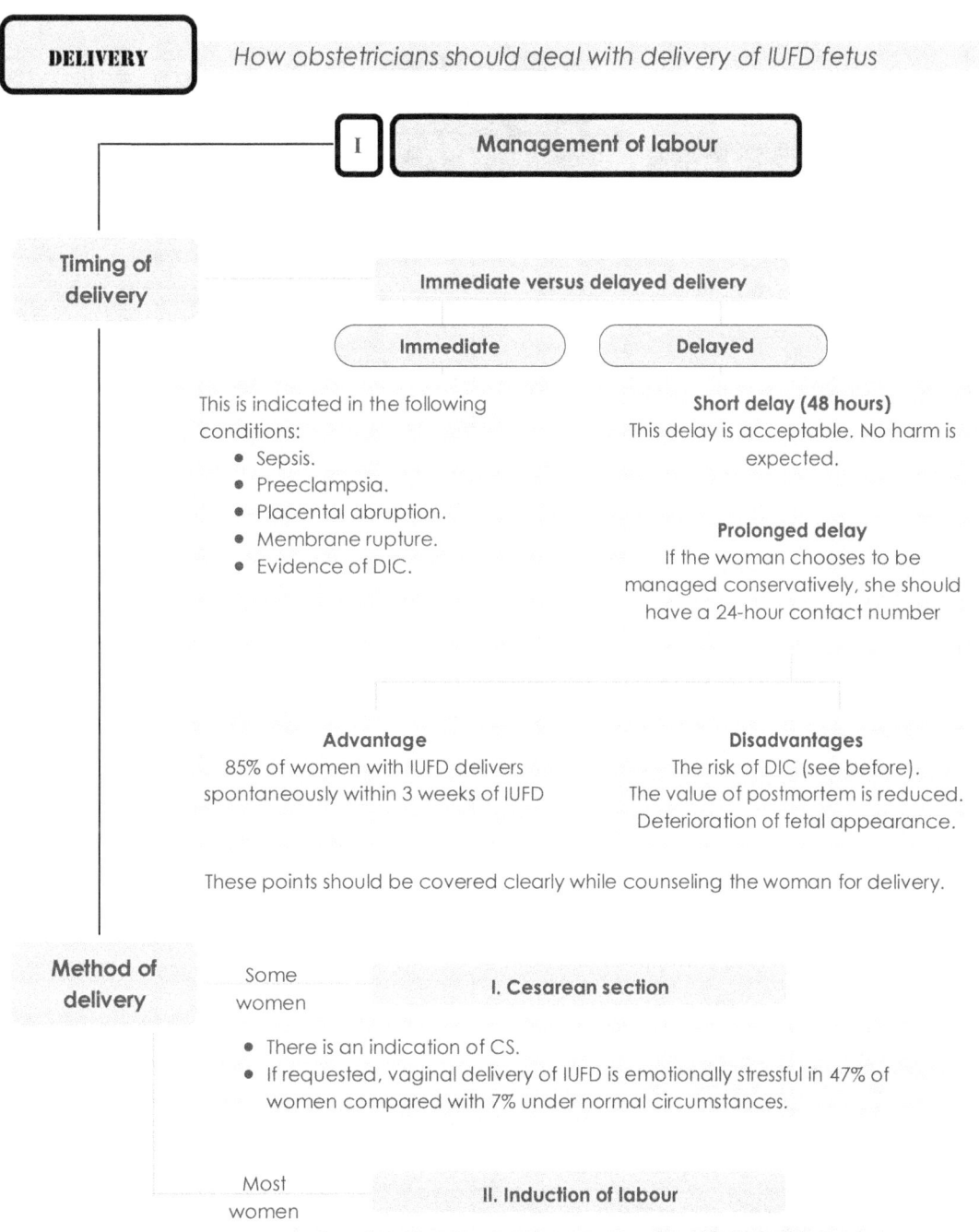

I   **Management of labour**

Timing of delivery

Immediate versus delayed delivery

Immediate   **Delayed**

This is indicated in the following conditions:
- Sepsis.
- Preeclampsia.
- Placental abruption.
- Membrane rupture.
- Evidence of DIC.

Short delay (48 hours)
This delay is acceptable. No harm is expected.

Prolonged delay
If the woman chooses to be managed conservatively, she should have a 24-hour contact number

Advantage
85% of women with IUFD delivers spontaneously within 3 weeks of IUFD

Disadvantages
The risk of DIC (see before).
The value of postmortem is reduced.
Deterioration of fetal appearance.

These points should be covered clearly while counseling the woman for delivery.

Method of delivery

Some women

I. Cesarean section

- There is an indication of CS.
- If requested, vaginal delivery of IUFD is emotionally stressful in 47% of women compared with 7% under normal circumstances.

Most women

II. Induction of labour

90% of women deliver within 24 hours of induction of labour

Facilities for IUFD labour
- Facilities for emergency care.
- A special labour ward room for uncomplicated IUFD (away from the sound of newborn s) with a nursing team trained to care with these women.
- A double bed room for the woman and her companion.
- Delivery by experienced midwife

Intrapartum antibiotic therapy
- IV broad-spectrum antibiotic therapy (including Chlamydia) is indicated in sepsis.
- Antibiotics are not given routinely or in GBS colonized women.
- Pyrexia secondary to prostaglandin use should be considered and misinterpreted as infection.

Pain relief during labour
- Diamorphine is recommended (in preference to pethidine).
- Regional anaesthesia can be offered. However, sepsis and DIC should be excluded before the procedure is offered (sepsis is associated with epidural abscess, DIC is associated with epidural and subdural hematoma).

Induction regimens for women with IUFD

Women with unscarred uterus

Mifepristone 200mg single dose *
PLUS

< 26 weeks	> 26 weeks
100 µg 6 hourly of misoprostol	25–50 µg 4-hourly of misoprostol

Misoprostol vs. prostaglandin E2
Misoprostol is a better choice (less cost, equal safety and efficacy).
Intra-vaginal misoprostol vs. IV oxytocin
Misoprostol is more effective than oxytocin.
Vaginal versus oral misoprostol
Vaginal misoprostol yields the same efficacy but with less side effects (nausea, vomiting, diarrhea, pyrexia)

Women with previous 2 CS

The risk of induction is slightly higher than in women with previous 1 CS

Women with > previous 2 CS

The safety of induction is unknown in these women

Women with previous CS should be monitored for the signs of scar dehiscence (maternal tachycardia, atypical pain, vaginal bleeding, haematuria and maternal collapse). The decision of oxytocin augmentation is made by the consultant

Women with previous LSCS

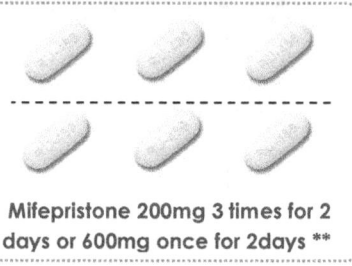

Mifepristone 200mg 3 times for 2 days or 600mg once for 2days **

OR

Trans-cervical balloon catheter (restricted to clinical trials)

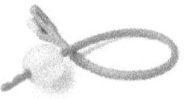

Advantages	Disadvantages
• 79% of women achieve vaginal birth. • Uterine rupture rate (0.58%) is lower than with prostaglandins (similar to spontaneous labour).	• There is increased risk of ascending infection in the presence of IUFD.

OR

Misoprostol

NICE recommends the use of lower doses (25–50 µg) for previous CS

Positives	Negatives
No evidence of an increased rate of hysterectomy or maternal death. Fetal distress risk is of no rule here	Higher risk of endometritis, blood transfusion and scar dehiscence and rupture (0.7%)

---

* Mifepristone (when added to misoprostol) reduces the time interval for labour by about 7 hours.
** This regimen increases the chance of labour within 72 hours (63% versus 17%.)

II	Postpartum management

Hospital stay

- A woman can return home immediately unless hospitalized for other medical inidciations.
- During hospital stay (if any), separate the woman from the maternity unit to avoid psychologic adverse effects.

Thrombo-prophylaxis

- IUFD is not a risk factor for thromboembolism. However, underlying etiologies of IUFD may indicate thromboprophylaxis.

Suppression of lactation

- **Dopamine agonists:** (90% effective).
  - *Bromocriptine:* 2.5 mg twice daily for 14 days.
  - *Cabergoline:* 1 mg (less rebound activity and side effects than bromocriptine). NEVER give these drugs to women with hypertension (including pre-eclampsia).
- **Other options:** non-pharmacological methods (e.g. support brassière, ice packs and analgesics) and estrogen are not suitable cohices.

Fertility - contraception

- The woman should be counseled about future fertility and contraception choice before leaving the hospital.
- The care provider should consider 2 points at that time:
  - Early conception following fetal loss may precipitate psychological problems.
  - Ovulation may return rapidly (18 days or later) due to suppression of lactation First menstrual period is not a good indictor of fertility return because before that, a woman is still exposed to pregnancy possibility.

Psychological support

Offer counseling to the woman, her partner and consider family members in this counseling. Advise couples about support groups.

Follow up — — — — — — Content of visits

- **First:** Discuss the results of previous investigations and the possible cause of IUFD. Give information about the chance of recurrence and how to avoid further loss.

- **Second:** Discuss delay of conception. The parents should be advised that delaying conception can give time for possible psychological sequences of IUFD to recover. However, both early pregnancy and delayed pregnancy can evoke anxiety.

- **Third:** Offer a pre-pregnancy advice regarding smoke cessation and optimization of body mass index (BMI).

| III | **Management in next pregnancy** |

During pregnancy

- Clear documentation of risk (previous IUFD).
- Women with a previous unexplained IUFD should be offered:
  - Obstetric antenatal care.
  - Screening for gestational diabetes.
- Women with previous IUFD (apparently normal but SGA) should be offered serial ultrasound assessment of growth.

During labour

- Woman with previous unexplained IUFD should deliver in specialist maternity unit.
- Woman with previous nonrecurrent cause of IUFD requires individual evaluation to choose for the place of birth.
- Scheduled birth should consider the gestational age of the previous IUFD, previous intrapartum events and induction of labour safety.

After labour

- After birth, women are at risk of depression. Risk factors for depression include:
  - Depression in the third trimester (risk extends up to 1 year after birth).
  - Women who conceive within < 12 months from a previous IUFD.
- Maternal bonding can be adversely affected.

Fact Box: Pregnancy following unexplained stillbirth

Women with a history of stillbirth (as a single risk) have:
- A 12-fold increased risk of intrapartum stillbirth.
- An increased risk of pre-eclampsia and placental abruption.
- An increased risk of gestational diabetes (four times).
- An increased risk of ischaemic placental disease, fetal distress, chorioamnionitis, extreme preterm birth and early neonatal mortality.

Appendix - I

Fetal and placental karyotyping

Written consent

It is necessary for any fetal samples

I. Tissue culture

Amniocentesis

A sample from the amniotic fluid may be used in women managed expectantly.

❶ Tissue sampling is taken from the deep fetal skin, cartilage and the placenta. Obtain several specimens to minimize the risk of failure.

❷ Preserve in a culture fluid that contains antibiotics to reduce the risk of bacterial contamination (culture failure).

❸ Keep culture bottles in the refrigerator away from formalin preservation bottles. They should be thawed slowly before examination.

❹ Genetic material should be stored if a single-gene syndrome is suspected.

If culture fails

II. QF-PCR

Quantitative fluorescent polymerase chain reaction (QF-PCR) can be performed on extracted DNA

Placental biopsy

Technique
Take approximately 1 cm from the fetal surface near cord insertion (to avoid maternal tissues).

Advantages
Placenta is the most viable tissue. It supplies rapid growing cells for tissue culture.

Disadvantages
Maternal contamination
Placental pseudomosaicism

Cartilage sample

It is the second choice. However, it is difficult to sample e.g. patella

Skin sample

Technique
Skin biopsy is taken deep to include underlying muscle (about 1 cm from the upper fleshy part of the thigh).

Disadvantages
Culture failure rate is ~60% (twice that of other tissues).

Tissue culture versus QF-PCR

Tissue culture	QF-PCR
Culture rovides wide range of genetic information (trisomies, monosomies, translocations, major deletions and marker chromosomes). Microdeletions are requested specifically based on postmortem examination findings.	It is reliable (<0.01% failure rate), efficient and cheap for aneuploidies. However, it is unreliable for the detection of translocations and marker chromosomes.

Appendix - II   **Postmortem examination**

Value of postmortem examination	• Postmortem examination of the baby and placenta is the most valuable diagnostic test. • Postmortem examination may identify the time of fetal death and may give information of medico-legal importance.

Counseling for postmortem	• Parents should be offered postmortem examination because this provides more information about the cause of IUFD and the management of next pregnancy. However, they should feel free to take their dicision. • Parents should be informed about what happens during the procedure and the possible appearance of the baby after the procedure. The parents should be reassured that their baby will be treated with dignity. • Written consent must be obtained for any invasive procedure under direct supervision (by an obstetrician or midwife trained in these consent issues and postmortem examination).

The consent (cover the following)
- The purpose of examination.
- The procedure and its extent.
- Possible organ/tissue retention and purpose.

Methods of postmortem examination

Placenta/cord

Pathological examination of the cord/placenta and membranes is recommended (even if not requested).

Medical imaging
- **Skeletal X-rays:** can show skeletal defects.
- **MRI:** for the brain and spinal cord (24% adds new information).
- **Ultrasound:** for internal organs (the value is not yet evaluated).

External examination

Examiner should report any apparent abnormalities, Weight and height should be reported (consider IUGR).

Autopsy/microscopy

Microscopic examination of relevant tissues should be performed (after parent's consent).

> **Levels of postmortem examination**

The level of postmortem examination goes down according to parent's request. However, the lower the level, the less conclusive the examination.

Full postmortem examination
The classic examination in the diagram

Limited postmortem examination
Restricted conventional postmortem examination

Limited postmortem examination
Minimally invasive examination

Disadvantages	Approach
• Its value is limited unless there is a specific suspicious organ that the parents agree to be examined. • It is technically difficult and may need more aggressive dissection than expected by the parents e.g. examination of the heart indicates removal of the lung and the thymus.	• **Minimally invasive surgical methods:** such as transcutaneous tissue biopsy, body-cavity aspiration (less informative). • **Medical imaging:** ultrasound and magnetic resonance imaging (MRI) are an adjuvant rather than a substitute for conventional postmortem.

Fact Box: Counseling before investigating the cause of IUFD

Certain points should be clear before investigating the cause of IUFD:

- No specific cause is found in almost half of stillbirths.
- Finding the cause can influence management of next pregnancy.
- Abnormal findings may not always be related to the cause of IUFD (e.g. factor V Leiden is present in 5% of population).
- Postmortem findings may necessitate further tests.

Appendix - III   **Sexing the lost baby**

Clinical examination

Examination of the external genitalia may be suspicious if the baby is severely macerated, extremely premature or massively hydropic. In these situations, 2 experienced healthcare practitioners (midwives, obstetricians, neonatologists or pathologists) should evaluate baby's genitalia.

If difficult or doubtful

Karyotyping

QF-PCR

Skin or placental tissue (even of macerated babies) can be tested using rapid karyotyping

FISH

Highly accurate results within 2 days

Fluorescence in situ hybridisation

If it fails

Tissue culture

Tissue culture takes longer time. Postmortem examination is also an option

Substitutes to baby sexing

If the genital sex cannot be definitely determined or if the parents do not wish for any postmortem examination. These options are still available:

- They can determine the sex themselves for registration. This can be helped by an ultrasound report or
- They can ask the midwife or doctor to determine sex.
- They can choose not to sex the baby and use a neutral name (registered as indeterminate sex).

Appendix - IV | **Medical certification of stillbirth (legal aspects)**

General rules

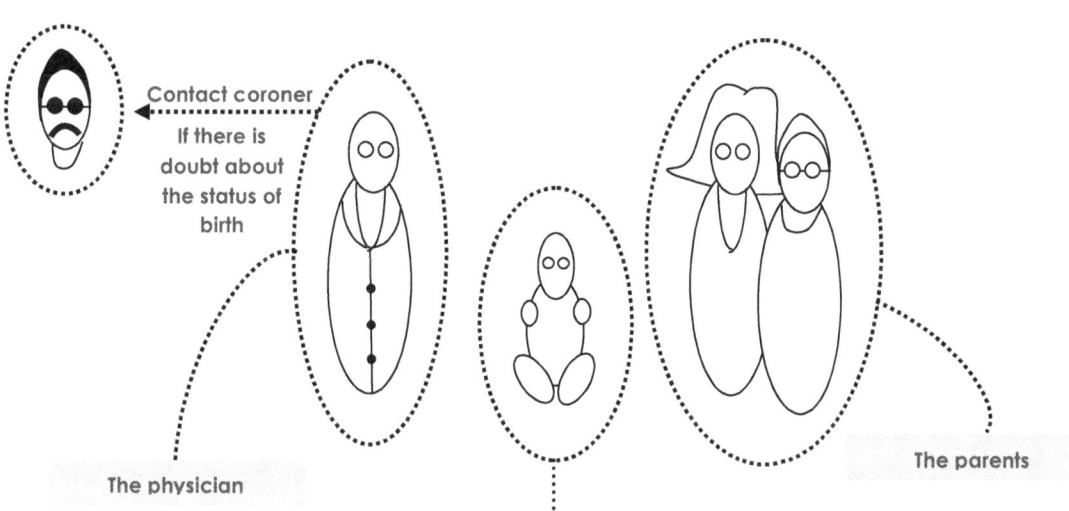

Contact coroner If there is doubt about the status of birth

The physician

A fully registered doctor or midwife who attends birth or examines the baby after birth should assign medical certificate of stillbirth.

Registration should include the cause and sequence of IUFD without using general terms e.g. anoxia, prematurity.

The baby

Only fetal deaths after 24 weeks need to be registered. If the baby is born after 24 weeks but is not is dead before completed 24 weeks of gestation, registration is not required.

The baby can be registered as indeterminate sex awaiting further tests.

The parents

Parents (the mother or the father if they were married at the time birth) are legally responsible for medical registration. However, they can delegate it to medical professional.

Timing for registration

Stillbirth should normally be registered within 42 days in UK (21 days in Scotland). The maximum time limit is 3 months (under exceptional conditions).

Registration data

The following data should be provided by the person in charge

- The place and date of birth of the baby
- The name and surname (If the parents wish)
- The sex of the baby (can be registered as indeterminate and later changed)
- The names, surnames, places of birth and occupations of the parents

- The mother's maiden name (if applicable)
- In Scotland, the marriage certificate of the parents is required.

If the couple were not married at the time of birth, the father's data is added only if:

- The mother and father go to the register office together or
- The father makes a statutory declaration of his paternity (the mother attends) or
- The mother makes a statutory declaration acknowledging the father's paternity (the father attends).

STATION 2: FETOLOGY

Red cell allo-immunization

BACKGROUND   *What obstetrician should basically know about red cell alloimmunization*

Pathogenesis

Red cell alloimmunization is an immune reaction that develops against foreign red cell antigens

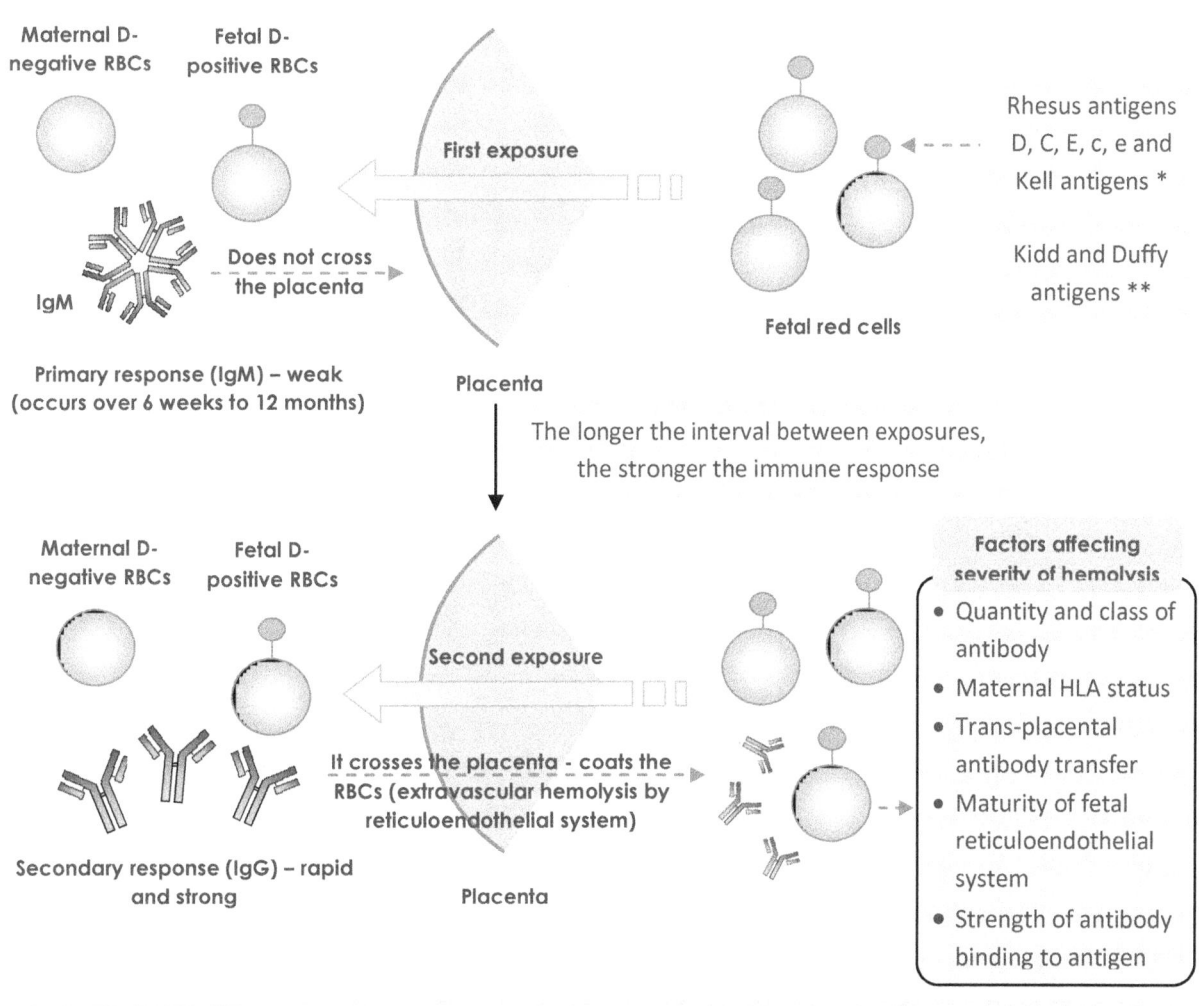

Maternal D-negative RBCs   **Fetal D-positive RBCs**

First exposure

Does not cross the placenta

IgM

Rhesus antigens D, C, E, c, e and Kell antigens *

Kidd and Duffy antigens **

Fetal red cells

Primary response (IgM) – weak (occurs over 6 weeks to 12 months)

Placenta

The longer the interval between exposures, the stronger the immune response

Maternal D-negative RBCs   **Fetal D-positive RBCs**

Second exposure

It crosses the placenta - coats the RBCs (extravascular hemolysis by reticuloendothelial system)

Secondary response (IgG) – rapid and strong

Placenta

Factors affecting severity of hemolysis
- Quantity and class of antibody
- Maternal HLA status
- Trans-placental antibody transfer
- Maturity of fetal reticuloendothelial system
- Strength of antibody binding to antigen

ABO system versus Rh incompatibility	• During intrauterine life, ABO antigens are weakly expressed. Rh antigens are strongly expressed by day 30. • Maternal-fetal ABO incompatibility reduces the risk of rhesus alloimmunisation

---

* Red cell antigens that commonly induce red cell alloimmunization and fetal hemolytic anaemia.

** Red cell antigens that commonly induce red cell alloimmunization

Pathogenesis (cont.)

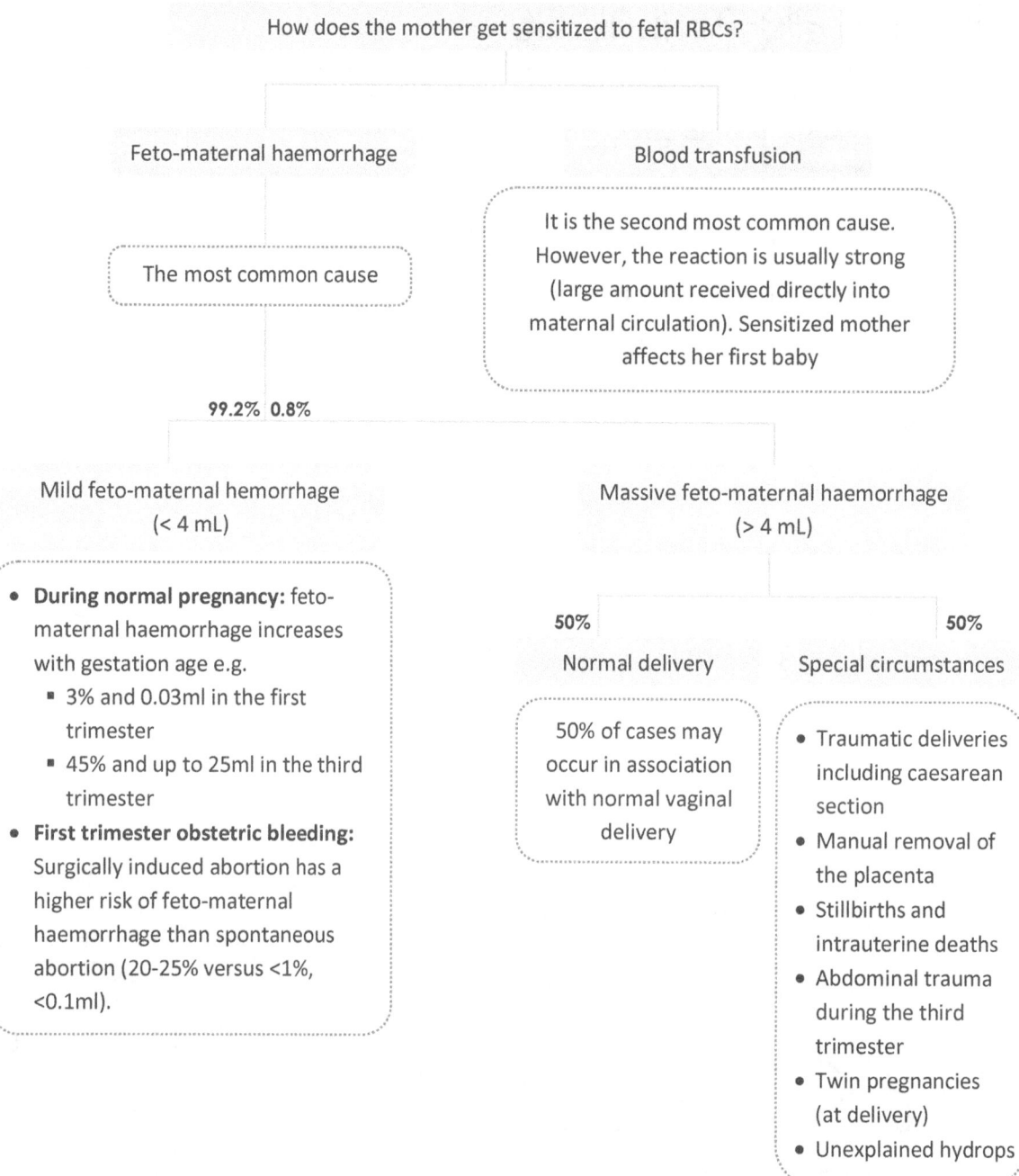

How does the mother get sensitized to fetal RBCs?

Feto-maternal haemorrhage

The most common cause

Blood transfusion

It is the second most common cause. However, the reaction is usually strong (large amount received directly into maternal circulation). Sensitized mother affects her first baby

99.2%   0.8%

Mild feto-maternal hemorrhage
(< 4 mL)

- **During normal pregnancy:** feto-maternal haemorrhage increases with gestation age e.g.
  - 3% and 0.03ml in the first trimester
  - 45% and up to 25ml in the third trimester
- **First trimester obstetric bleeding:** Surgically induced abortion has a higher risk of feto-maternal haemorrhage than spontaneous abortion (20-25% versus <1%, <0.1ml).

Massive feto-maternal haemorrhage
(> 4 mL)

50%   **50%**

Normal delivery   Special circumstances

50% of cases may occur in association with normal vaginal delivery

- Traumatic deliveries including caesarean section
- Manual removal of the placenta
- Stillbirths and intrauterine deaths
- Abdominal trauma during the third trimester
- Twin pregnancies (at delivery)
- Unexplained hydrops

APPROACH   *How obstetricians should deal with these cases in a stepwise manner*

Management of red cell alloimmunization depends on the state of immunization of the mother and the presence of previous history of fetal hydrops. It also depends on the red cell antigen system involved (Rhesus versus non-rhesus alloimmunization).

I | **Women with D allo-immunization**

Initial assessment

| Possibly Immunized women (second pregnancy) | Non-immunized Rh negative women (first pregnancy) | Immunized women with history of fetal hemolysis |

Determination of maternal Rh status in the first antenatal visit

If Rhesus is negative

Determination of paternal Rh status (paternal blood, CVS or amniocentesis or free fetal DNA in maternal serum)

| **Positive** | **Negative** |

| Antibody screening (indirect Coombs test) | No further management needed |

At screening and every 4 weeks from the 20th weeks)

Determination of anti-D titer

| Anti-D > 10 IU/mL (or 1:8 -1:32) | Anti-D 4-10 IU/mL | Anti-D < 4 IU/mL (or ≤ 1:8) | Give ant-D serum at 28 weeks (± second dose at 34 weeks) |

| Follow up monthly | Follow up every 2 weeks | Middle cerebral artery Doppler peak systolic velocity | |

| | If normal | If close to abnormal | If abnormal (> 1.5 MoM) |

| If normal | Repeat every 2 weeks | Repeat every 1 week | Interference |

| | | **≥ 35 weeks** | **< 35 weeks** |

| Follow up until 37-38 weeks | **Delivery** | | **Intrauterine transfusion** |

| | Give steroids and deliver at 32-34 weeks | | Done every 2 weeks, last one at 30-32 weeks |

| II | Women with non-D allo-immunization |

All women

Testing for anti-C, anti-c, anti-E and anti-K1 (Kell) antibodies at booking

History of fetal haemolysis

Refer before 20 weeks of gestation

Negative

Repeat routinely at the 28th week

Low titer

< 1:32 (< 7.5 IU/ml for anti-c and < 1:8 for anti-Kell)

High titer   Or positive Kell

Determine paternal antigenic state

Repeat every 4 weeks until 28 weeks then every 2 weeks

Positive

Determine paternal zygosity

Negative

No further screening required

Delivery at 37-38 weeks

Homozygous

Weekly middle cerebral artery Doppler peak systolic velocity is indicated after 18 weeks of gestation

Heterozygous

Amniocentesis or free fetal DNA in maternal blood for fetal antigen typing (E, C, c, K1)

Negative

Positive

Normal

If < 1.5 MoM, repeat every 1 week

Abnormal

If > 1.5 MoM, manage according to gestational age

Delivery

> 35 weeks

< 35 weeks

Delivery can be postponed until 37-38 weeks, or immediate delivery is allowed for a mature fetus if complications develop during transfusion

Intrauterine transfusion

Non-D red cell antibodies

Anti-Kell antibodies

- Among the 24 types of this antigen, 8 can cause fetal haemolysis. The most common are KEL 1 and KEL2 (the incidence is only 0.1-0.2%).
- The antigen is more common is white than black population (9% versus 2%). It is also more commonly heterozygous in black than white (100% versus 97.8%).
- Anti-Kell antibodies differ from anti-D antibodies in the following:
  - It is most commonly caused by blood transfusion. However, the response to transfusion is less severe than that induced by previous pregnancy.
  - Previous history of Kell alloimmunization does not always predict the outcome of next pregnancy.

Anti-c antibodies

- 14–21% of c-positive babies born to mothers with anti-c required exchange transfusion.
- Generally, 80% of males are c-positive (60% being heterozygous with 50% of fetuses affected).
- The risk of haemolysis is related to anti-c titre:
  - **7.5 iu/ml:** low risk - continue to monitor.
  - **7.5–20 iu/ml or titre (1:32):** risk of moderate haemolysis.
  - **> 20 iu/ml:** Risk of severe haemolysis.
- Anti-c may cause delayed anaemia in the neonate.

Anti-E antibodies

- 40% of people with anti-c also contain anti-E.
- Anti-E can be either:
  - **natural IgM:** without immune stimulation or
  - **IgG:** in women with a history of transfusion or previous pregnancy.
- Fetal haemolysis is mild in 77% of cases (severe in 10% of cases).

Duffy antibodies

- The Duffy antigen system consists of two antigens: Fya and Fyb.
- Antibody titre levels is not related with fetal outcome.

Kidd antibodies

- The Kidd antigen system consists of two antigens: Jka and Jkb.
- They are usually associated with mild haemolysis.

ABO antibodies

- ABO antibodies are a rare cause of hemolytic disease of the newborn and the disease is generally mild.
- Haemolytic disease of the fetus and newborn caused by ABO antibodies affects almost only fetuses of group O mothers by the action of anti-A and anti-B IgG antibodies.

PROPHYLAXIS   *What are the recent recommendations for using the anti-D serum*

What is the anti-D serum

- Anti-D Ig is extracted from the plasma of donors who have high circulating levels of anti-D produced by deliberate immunisation of Rh-negative donors.
- As a protective measure, specific virology testing is performed to test the donors then and the product undergoes a viral inactivation process.

Types of anti-D serum

Type	Dose	Route
D-GAM	250, 500, 1500, 2500 iu	IM only *
Partobulin SDF	1250 iu (prefilled syringe)	IM only
Rhophylac	1500 iu (prefilled syringe)	IM and IV
WinRho SDF	1500and 5000 IU (vials)	IM and IV

* IM injection is better in the deltoid muscle (gluteal injection usually reach the subcutaneous tissue)

The dose of anti-D serum

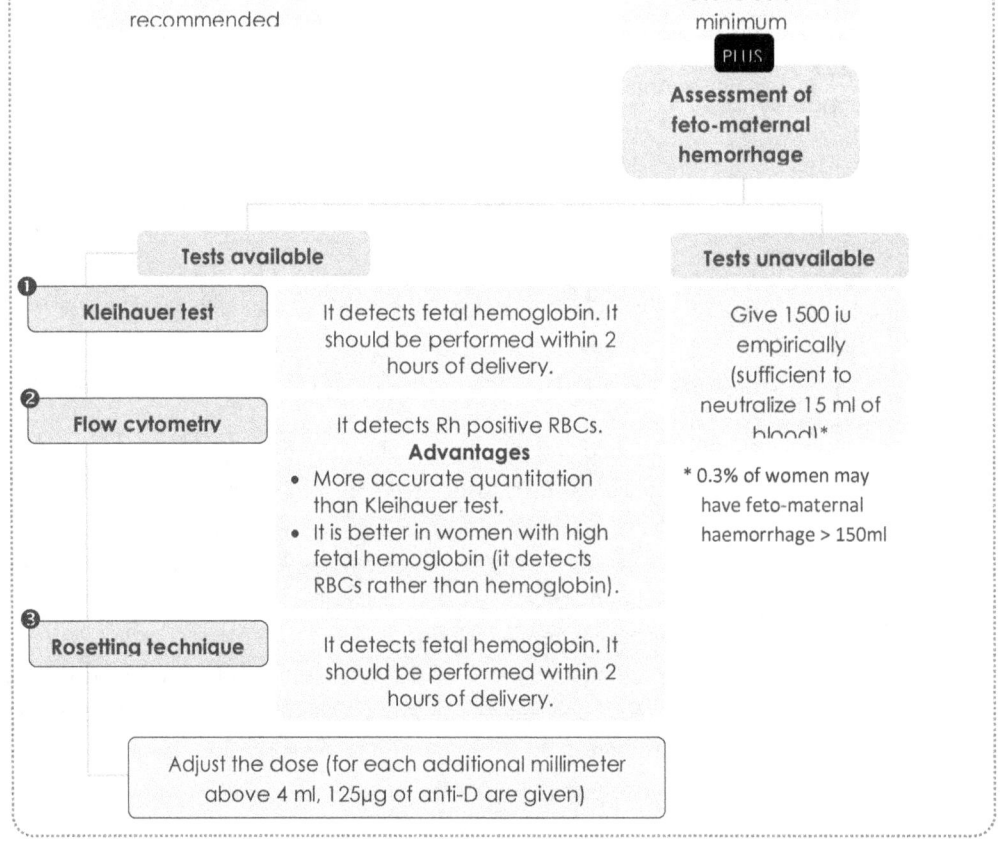

Gestational age

< 20 weeks

250 iu is recommended

≥ 20 weeks

500 iu as a minimum

PLUS

Assessment of feto-maternal hemorrhage

Tests available

① **Kleihauer test** — It detects fetal hemoglobin. It should be performed within 2 hours of delivery.

② **Flow cytometry** — It detects Rh positive RBCs.
Advantages
- More accurate quantitation than Kleihauer test.
- It is better in women with high fetal hemoglobin (it detects RBCs rather than hemoglobin).

③ **Rosetting technique** — It detects fetal hemoglobin. It should be performed within 2 hours of delivery.

Adjust the dose (for each additional millimeter above 4 ml, 125µg of anti-D are given)

Tests unavailable

Give 1500 iu empirically (sufficient to neutralize 15 ml of blood)*

* 0.3% of women may have feto-maternal haemorrhage > 150ml

The time of administration
- Anti-D Ig should be given as soon as possible after the sensitising event. In general, it should always be given within 72 hours.
- If it is not given before 72 hours, it should also be given soon because the dose can still be of some benefit up to 10 days after the event.

Route of administration
- **Subcutaneous or intramuscular route:** D-GAM, Partobulin SDF.
- **Intravenous or intramuscular route:** Rophylac, WinRho SDF.

The subcutaneous route is recommended in women with bleeding tendency.

Sensitizing events

 Obstetric events

Miscarriage
- Anti-D Ig is not indicated in RhD-negative women with *spontaneous miscarriage* before 12 weeks of gestation.
- Anti-D Ig is indicated for all non-sensitised RhD-negative women who have a *spontaneous miscarriage* (complete or incomplete) at or after 12 weeks of gestation.
- Anti-D Ig is indicated in non-sensitised RhD-negative women managed with *medical or surgical evacuation* of the uterus regardless of gestation.
- Anti-D Ig is indicated in all non-sensitised RhD-negative women with *a threatened miscarriage* after 12 weeks of gestation (or approaching 12 weeks with heavy or repeated bleeding or associated abdominal pain). If bleeding continues intermittently after 12 weeks of gestation, anti-D Ig should be given every 6 weeks.

Ectopic pregnancy

Anti-D Ig is indicated in all non-sensitised RhD-negative women who have an ectopic pregnancy (regardless of management).

Other events

These events indicate anti-D Ig administration regardless of any routine doses given):
- Invasive prenatal diagnosis (amniocentesis, chorion villus sampling, cordocentesis, intrauterine transfusion).
- Other intrauterine procedures (e.g. insertion of shunts, embryo reduction, laser)
- Antepartum haemorrhage
- External cephalic version of the fetus (including attempted)
- Any abdominal trauma (direct/indirect, sharp/blunt, open/closed)
- Fetal death.

❷ Non-obstetric events

Rh D-positive platelet transfusion

- Non-sensitized Rh negative women receiving RhD-positive platelets should be given prophylaxis against Rh alloimmunisation. Each unit of platelets contains < 0.1 ml red cells.
- 250 iu (50 micrograms) anti-D Ig should be given subcutaneously following every 3 adult doses of platelets.

Rh D-positive blood transfusion

- **When < 15 ml of RhD-positive blood is transfused:** to an RhD-negative woman, anti-D Ig should be given (500 iu of anti-D Ig per each 4 ml of blood).
- **When > 15 ml is transfused:** larger anti-D Ig intramuscular preparation (2500 iu or 5000 iu) is recommended.
- **When > 2 units of RhD-positive blood are transfused:** an exchange transfusion (after counseling) is recommended to reduce the antigen load and the dose of anti-D Ig needed.

Following immunization particularly in large doses, passive anti-D Igs given may be detected in the circulation for up to 6 months. Accordingly, testing for immune anti-D cannot be conclusive before 9-12 months.

Appendix - I   **Routine antenatal anti-D prophylaxis (RAADP)**

| **What is the RAADP system?** | RAADP refers to antenatal anti-D Ig administration to all non-sensitised RhD-negative women apart from doses given in response to potentially sensitising events. |

What is the rationale of RAADP?

- Silent sensitization (without sensitizing accidents) occurs in < 10% before 28 weeks of gestation but the incidence increases with advancing gestational age to 55-80%. RAADP prevents this silent sensitisation and its possible sequences.
- In the absence of RAADP, 1% of RhD-negative women with an RhD-positive baby will be sensitised.

RAADP protocol

- Before receiving anti-D serum, an informed decision should be made and consent recorded in the case notes. Written information should be supplied to help making a proper decision.
- Routine 28-week antibody screening is made before the first dose of anti-D is given.
- There are two regimens for providing RAADP:
    1. Two doses of 500 iu anti-D Ig at 28 and 34 weeks of gestation or
    2. A single dose of 1500 iu at 28 weeks of gestation.
  There are no evidence that one regimen is superior to the other.
- After immunization, passive anti-D Igs can be detected for up to 8 weeks or more, and is ≤ 1 iu/ml. Accurate documentation of anti-D Ig is thus essential.

Maternal/ fetal effects of RAADP?

There is no evidence of any adverse events to the mother or baby. The only risk is the possibility of blood-borne infection, and procedures are in place to minimise risks.

Declining RAADP

- If RAADP is declined after proper counseling, this should be documented in the case notes with the reasons for the decision.
- Some causes of decline include:
    1. women who object on religious grounds.
    2. women who will be sterilised after birth.
    3. women who are certain they will have no more children.
    4. women who are in a stable relationship with the genetic father of their children and the father is known or found to be RhD-negative.
- If RAADP is declined, antibody screening should be performed at booking and at 28 weeks of gestation to identify if sensitisation has occurred.

Fact Box: anti-D serum

- Anti-D serum does not protect against the development of other antibodies.
- Women who have weak expression of Rh-D (Du) do not form anti-D antibodies and do not require prophylaxis.

Appendix - II   **Invasive procedures in HDFN* management**

Amniocentesis

- Amniocentesis is carried out to obtain a sample from the amniotic fluid. This sample is analyzed using spectophotometry to estimate bilirubin level (OD450) as an indirect indicator of haemolysis and fetal anaemia. This measurement is plotted on Liley's chart.

  If the measures are blotted in zone 3 or increasing in zone 2, this indicates severe haemolysis and is an indication for termination of pregnancy if the fetus is mature or intrauterine transfusion if the fetus is preterm.
- Amniocentesis is unreliable before 28 weeks gestation. It is also unreliable in Kell disease
- Amniocentesis has been replaced by middle cerebral artery peak systolic velocity using Doppler.

Cordocentesis

- Cordocentesis is made to directly estimate fetal hemoglobin. Severe anaemia is considered if hematocrite value < 30%.
- Both amniocentesis and cordocentesis carry the risk of fetal loss (1-2% per procedure) and the risk of feto-maternal haemorrhage and increased maternal antibody level.

Intra-uterine transfusion

- Intrauterine transfusion is done using packed O sero-negative red cells compatible with both the mother and fetus. A local anaesthetic is applied at the site of needle insertion along with antiseptic solution.
- Ultrasound is used to guide the needle through the mother's abdomen into the fetus's abdomen (intra-peritoneal) or an umbilical cord vein (better).
- Transfusion of blood that achieves supranormal Hb concentration allows longer interval between transfusions (2-4 weeks).
- Procedure-related fetal loss rate is 2-4%
- Delivery after 34 weeks gestation may be considered safer than continued intra-uterine transfusion (last transfusion is done at 30-32 weeks).

Treatment options that aim at eradicating maternal anti-D antibodies such as plasmapheresis and maternal intravenous immune globulin have limited efficacy.

---

* HDFN = Haemolytic disease of the fetus and the newborn

STATION 2: FETOLOGY

Fetal hydrops

BACKGROUND *What obstetrician should basically know about fetal hydrops*

What is fetal hydrops

This term refers to the presence of generalised fetal edema with accumulation of fluid within 2 or more body cavities (ascites, pleural effusion, pericardial effusions and polyhydramnios).

Causes of fetal hydrops

Immune hydrops

> Immune hydrops is associated with anti - D Rhesus antibodies, antibodies to K (Kell), antibodies to Fya (Duffy)

Heart

> Severe congenital heart disease
> Cardiac arrhythmias (e.g. paroxysmal supraventricular tachycardia resulting in heart failure)
> Premature closure of ductus arteriosus

Chest

> Intra-thoracic tumors
> cystic adenomatoid malformation of the lung (CAML)
> Extralobar pulmonary sequestration
> Pulmonary hypoplasia
> Diaphragmatic hernia

Abdomen

> Lower urinary tract anomalies
> Intra-abdominal tumours e.g. ovarian cysts

Others

> Placental chorioangioma
> Sacro-coccygeal terratoma

Non-immune hydrops

30% of cases are idiopathic

Structural anomalies

Non-structural anomalies

Anaemia

Hemolytic
Homozygous α-thalassaemia
G6PD deficiency
Pyruvate kinase deficiency
Lethal hereditary spherocytosis
Diamond-Blackfan syndrome (Inherited erythroblastopenia)
Secondary
Twin to twin transfusion syndrome
Chronic FMH

Aneuploidy

Trisomies
Turner syndrome
Triploidy

Metabolism

lysosomal storage disease e.g. beta-glucuronidase deficiency and generalised gangliosidosis

Infection

Viruses
Parvovirus B19
Cytomegalovirus
Herpes simplex
Hepatitis B
Adenovirus
Coxsackievirus B
Spirocheates
Syphilis
Leptospirosis
Parasites
Toxoplasmosis
Chagas disease
Bacteria
Listeria
Ureaplasma

CHAPTER 3
EARLY PREGNANCY COMPLICATIONS

STATION 3: EARLY OBSTETRIC COMPLICATIONS

Early pregnancy loss & Miscarriage

BACKGROUND — *What obstetrician should basically know about early pregnancy loss*

Definitions

Term	Definition
Miscarriage	Pregnancy loss under 24 weeks of gestation
Empty sac	Sac with absent or minimal structures
Fetal loss	Previous CRL measurement with subsequent loss of fetal heart activity
Biochemical pregnancy loss	Pregnancy not located on scan
Early pregnancy loss (delayed miscarriage)	An empty sac or sac with no fetal heart activity less than 12 weeks
Late pregnancy loss	Loss of fetal heart activity > 12 weeks
Pregnancy of unknown location	Positive hCG with no identifiable pregnancy on ultrasound scan

Types of miscarriage

Term	Old term
Threatened miscarriage	Threatened abortion
Inevitable miscarriage	Inevitable abortion
Incomplete miscarriage	Incomplete abortion
Complete miscarriage	Inevitable abortion
Missed miscarriage	Missed abortion
Recurrent miscarriage	Recurrent abortion
Early fetal demise	Blighted ovum – anembryonic pregnancy
Miscarriage with sepsis	Septic abortion

The term MISCARRIAGE is now recommended instead of other terms e.g. incompetent cervix, failure of pregnancy which may have adverse impact on the mother. Miscarriage represents 10-20% of clinical pregnancies

APPROACH *How obstetricians should deal with early pregnancy loss*

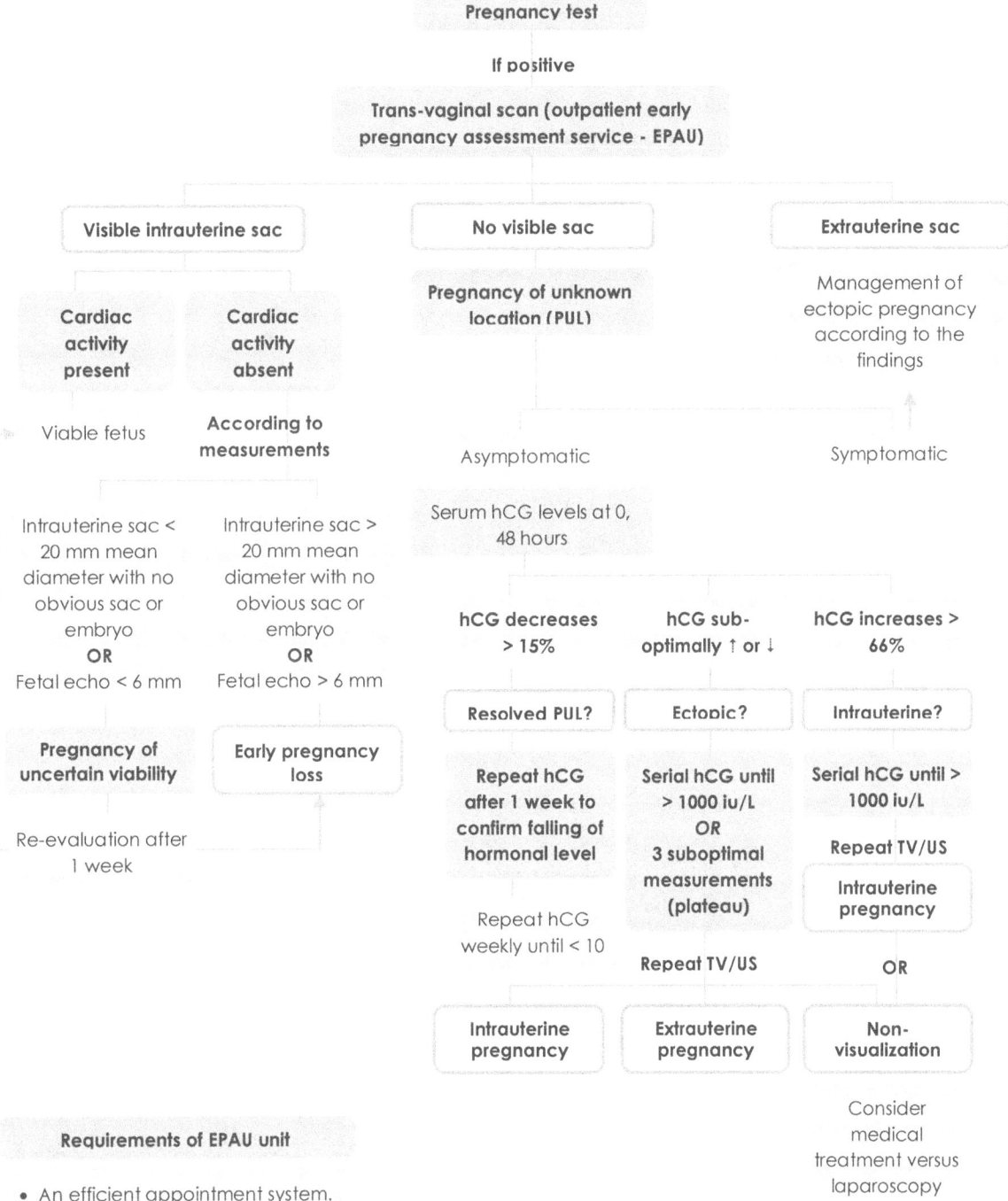

Requirements of EPAU unit

- An efficient appointment system.
- Suitable Ultrasound equipment.
- Laboratory facilities for rhesus antibody testing, hCG and progesterone.
- Available information leaflets, referral and discharge letters.

Pregnancy test

- **Urinary HCG:** urine-based hCG test is used by the majority of women. Monoclonal antibody based kits can detect hCG at 25 iu/l (Day 9 postconception or day 23 of a 28-day cycle).
- **Serum HCG:** it provides quantative measurement of the hormone.

Trans-vaginal ultrasound

Early trans-vaginal ultrasound is carried out following a positive pregnancy test. Possible findings are:

- **Definite intrauterine sac:** the incidence of pregnancy of uncertain viability in the first EPAU visit is 10%.

  If the sac is empty, it is important that the sonographer should record whether the sac is eccentrically placed in the fundus (suggesting intrauterine pregnancy) or centrally placed with a double-ring pattern (suggesting extrauterine pregnancy).

- **Extrauterine pregnancy:** management is ectopic pregnancy is made according to clinical circumstances.
- **No visible sac:** the incidence of pregnancy of unknown location is 8-10%.

Serial hCG assessment

On follow up, these patterns can be identified:

- **The discriminatory zone:** it refers to the level of hCG at which pregnancy should be visualized by trans-vaginal scan. Absence of gestational sac at this level indicates extra-uterine pregnancy.
- **Doubling time:** the normal doubling of hCG titer is 48 hours. However, in twin pregnancy or heterotopic pregnancy, a suboptimal rise may be misleading.
- **Titer plateau below 1000 iu/l:** The possible outcomes are:
  - Pregnancy of unknown location.
  - Miscarriage.
  - Gestational trophoblastic disease.
  - Cranial germ cell tumour.

  The last 2 possibilities are rare and serum hCG levels are likely to be greater than 1000 iu/l.

Serum progesterone

Serum progesterone can be used in conjunction with ultrasound in women with pregnancy of unknown location.

Level	Interpretation
Above 60 nmol/l	Strongly associated with normal intrauterine pregnancy
Above 25 nmol/l	Mostly associated with normal intrauterine pregnancy
Below 25 nmol/l	Usually associated with non-viable pregnancy
Below 20 nmol/l	Usually associated with spontaneous resolution
Below 15.9 nmol/l	Some cases of viable pregnancy are still reported *

* Accordingly, uterine evacuation should be made based on low initial progesterone.

Management of pregnancy loss

IF

- Persistent excessive bleeding.
- Haemodynamic instability.
- Infected retained tissue.
- Suspected gestational trophoblastic disease.

- Incomplete miscarriage.
- Early fetal demise at gestations < 71 days or
- Sac diameter less than 24mm *

- Confirmed first-trimester miscarriage particularly incomplete miscarriage
- Woman's acceptance of possible long expectancy.

Counseling

Surgical uterine evacuation

Medical uterine evacuation

Expectant management

Pre-abortion evaluation

Determination of Rh status

When clinically indicated: test for blood grouping, haemoglobin, haemoglobinpathies, red cell antibodies

Venous thromboembolism risk assessment

Cervical cytology is offered to women who do not follow the screening schedule (or give advice about screening)

Venous thromboembolism risk assessment

Screening for Chlamydia infection and risk assessment of other STIs. Give information about STI prevention

Antibiotic prophylaxis against Chlamydia trachomatis and anaerobes for both surgical abortion (evidence grade: A) and medical abortion (evidence grade: C)

Discuss appropriate contraception plan following abortion

Pre-abortion evaluation

Wait for spontaneous resorption. Women should be able to access 24-hour telephone advice and emergency admission if required.

If persistent excessive bleeding develops

Anti-D serum not indicated < 12 weeks

Surgical uterine evacuation

* There is no difference in the success rate of surgical versus medical evacuation in these indications. Acceptability is equal in both methods. Medical evacuation has lower risk of pelvic infection.

Procedure (Surgical)

Cervical preparation	Pain relief and anaesthesia
< 14 weeks Misoprostol 400 µg vaginally 3 hours or sublingually 2-3 hours prior to surgery **14-18 weeks** Osmotic dilators (best) or misoprostol	**Anaesthesia** General anaesthesia versus conscious sedation (woman choice) **Analgesia** NSAIDs are given during surgical abortion (routinely).

< 7 weeks	8-14 weeks	14-16 weeks	> 14 weeks
Vacuum aspiration – Aspirate should be examined	Vacuum aspiration (electric or manual)	Vacuum aspiration – Aspirate should be examined	D & E under ultrasound guidance

Histopathology	**Anti-D serum**
Not indicated as a routine	For Rh non-sensitized women (within 72 hrs)

Procedure (Medical)

Pain relief

NSAIDs are given during medical abortion. Some women may need narcotics (particularly after 13 weeks of gestation)

Incomplete miscarriage	Missed miscarriage

Give the usual dose of misoprostol alone

< 7 weeks
Mifepristone 200 mg orally → 24-48 hours later → Misoprostol 800 µg vaginal, buccal or sublingual

7-9 weeks
Mifepristone 200 mg orally → 24-48 hours later → Misoprostol 400 µg
Repeat if no response within 4 hours

9-13 weeks
Mifepristone 200 mg orally → 36-48 hours later → Misoprostol 800 µg
Misoprostol 400 µg every 3 hours (maximum 4 times)

13-24 weeks
Mifepristone 200 mg orally → 36-48 hours later → Misoprostol 800 µg
No response after 3 hours – repeat mifepristone – misoprostol after 12 hours
Misoprostol 400 µg every 3 hours (maximum 4 times)

Fact Box: surgical uterine evacuation

- Early vacuum aspiration (< 7 weeks) should be confirmed by examination of the aspirate to confirm gestation.
- Aspiration should not be completed by sharp curettage or ultrasound guidance.

Counseling

Counseling before surgical evacuation

Before surgical evacuation, women should be counseled that the incidence of serious morbidity is 2.1% (mortality of 0.5/100 000). Blood transfusion, laparoscopy or laparotomy may be indicated. The causes of morbidity (complications) are:
- Perforation.
- Cervical tears.
- Intraabdominal trauma.
- Intrauterine adhesions.
- Haemorrhage.

Counseling before medical evacuation

20% of women prefer medical evacuation to avoid general anaesthesia and to be more in control. However, women should be informed that:
- Bleeding may continue for up to 3 weeks after medical evacuation.
- Success rate varies from 13% to 96% depending on:
  - The type of miscarriage (highest if incomplete).
  - Sac size.
  - Whether follow-up is clinical or involves ultrasound (highest with clinical rather ultrasound follow up).
  - Total dose (highest with high dose misoprostol "1200-1400 µg").
  - Duration of use and route of administration of prostaglandin (highest with vaginal route).

Counseling before expectant management

- Women should be informed that complete resolution may take several weeks and is often followed by minimal bleeding. The overall success rates are lower. Factors affecting success are:
  - The type of miscarriage.
  - Duration of follow-up.
  - Whether ultrasound or clinical assessment.
  - A low serum progesterone level (predicts pregnancy that may tend to resolve spontaneously).
- Woman should be informed that the passage of tissue may be associated with heavy bleeding that may indicate surgical evacuation.

Ultrasound criteria used to define 'retained products' varies between studies (generally < 50 mm).

Complications of abortion (general counseling)

General complications

- **Severe bleeding requiring transfusion:**
  - The risk in early abortions is < 1 in 1000.
  - The risk beyond 20 weeks is 4 in 1000.
- **Uterine perforation (surgical abortion only):**
  The risk is 1-4 in 1000 (depending on gestational age and experience).
- **Cervical trauma (surgical abortion only):**
  The risk of damage to the external os is 1 in 100 or less (depending on gestational age and experience).
- **Uterine rupture (medical abortion at late gestations):**
  The risk is < 1 in 1000.

Failed abortion

The risk of failure of abortion is < 1:100. Women should be counseled that surgical evacuation following failed medical abortion or re-evacuation following surgical procedure is indicated in less than 5% of cases.

Post-abortion infection

Post-abortion infection is usually an outcome of pre-existing genital infection. Woman should be informed that genital screening and prophylactic antibiotics can reduce the risk.

Preterm birth

The risk of preterm labour increases slightly with induced abortion. The risk increases with the number of abortions. However, the evidence of causality is not yet proven.

Psychological complications

Women with unintended pregnancy usually do not suffer psychological complications unless there is history of mental health problems. Proper history taking and counseling are essential.

Induced abortion is not associated with breast cancer. There is no evidence with association with adverse reproductive outcomes

Antibiotic therapy

Regimen 1

Azithromycin 1 g orally on the day of abortion, plus metronidazole 1 g rectally or 800 mg orally prior to or at the time of abortion

Regimen 2

Doxycycline 100 mg orally twice daily for 7 days, starting on the day of the abortion, plus metronidazole 1 g rectally or 800 mg orally prior to or at the time of the abortion

Regimen 3

Metronidazole 1 g rectally or 800 mg orally prior to or at the time of abortion for women who have tested negative for C. trachomatis infection.

Post-treatment care

Information after abortion

- Written information about the procedure is provided at the time of discharge (to allow other practitioners to manage any complications).
- Written (& verbal) information about possible symptoms related to complications or failed abortion should be provided.
- A 24 hour telephone number should be provided for help.

Anti-D serum

Contraception

Discuss future contraceptive method. Initiate immediately if possible. Intrauterine device can be inserted if abortion is confirmed to be complete. Sterilization is also possible before discharge.

Follow up after abortion

- If abortion is confirmed to be complete at the time of the procedure, there is no need for routine follow up visits. Follow up visits should be allowed according to woman's wish.
- In case of doubt, follow up is indicated (clinical follow up rather than routine sonogrpahic examination). Clinical findings are the base of re-evacuation decision.

Fact Box: Induced abortion

- Induced abortion in women with viable pregnancy should be offered feticide. She should be counseled about the use of ultrasound.
- Form HSA1 (Certificate A in Scotland) is completed by the doctor in the abortion service unit if a woman refers herself, or if her doctor does not support abortion.
- Abortion service should be provided without delay. This includes:
  - Referral to an abortion service within 2 working days.
  - Abortion service assessment within 5 working days of referral or self-referral.
  - Abortion procedure within 5 working days of the decision to proceed.
  - The total time from seeing the abortion provider to the procedure should not exceed 10 working days.
  - The procedure is made as soon as possible in the presence of medical indication.
- Medical abortion (misoprostol) up to 9 weeks of gestation can be discharged.

Appendix — Abortion: Related legal issues

The Abortion Act

- The Abortion Act 1967 (amended by the Human Fertilisation and Embryology Act 1990) is applied in England, Scotland and Wales.
- Abortion act provides the legal requirements of certification and notification of abortion procedures.
- This requirements include:
  - An abortion requires 2 registered medical practitioners to agree (in good faith) that an abortion is justified within the terms of the Act.
  - Only a registered medical practitioner (doctor) can terminate a pregnancy. However, a nurse or midwife may administer the drugs prescribed by the doctor for medical abortion once these have been prescribed by a doctor.

Abortion forms

Doctors are obligated to complete these forms

HSA1 — It is the certificate of opinion regarding abortion under section 1(1). This form is signed by 2 doctors. This form must be kept for 3 years.

HSA2 — It is the certificate of emergency abortion. It is completed by the doctor (rather than 2 in HSA1) within 24 hours of emergency abortion. This form must be kept for 3 years.

HSA4 — It is the form to be sent to the Chief Medical Officer (CMO) either manually or electronically (electronic notification is not available in Scotland). It is completed by the doctor who terminated pregnancy and is sent within 14 days (7 days in Scotland).

Statutory grounds

Abortion should be based on 1 or more of the grounds specified in the Abortion Act

A	Continuance of pregnancy endangers the life of the pregnant woman greater than if the pregnancy is terminated.	Section 1(1)(c)
B	Continuance of pregnancy can lead to grave permanent injury to the physical or mental health of the pregnant woman.	Section 1(1)(b)
C	Continuance of pregnancy can involve injury to the physical or mental health of the pregnant woman. Pregnancy is less than 24 weeks of gestation.	Section 1(1)(a)
D	Continuance of pregnancy can involve injury to the physical or mental health of any child(ren) of the family of the woman. Pregnancy is less than 24 week.	Section 1(1)(a)
E	There is a risk of physical or mental abnormalities to the born child as to be seriously handicapped.	Section 1(1)(d)
F	Emergency procedure to save the life of the pregnant woman	Section 1(4)
G	Emergency procedure to prevent permanent injury to the pregnant woman	

* HSA1 (Certificate A in Scotland) – HAS2 (Certificate B in Scotland)

STATION 3: EARLY OBSTETRIC COMPLICATIONS

Recurrent miscarriage

BACKGROUND *What obstetrician should basically know about recurrent miscarriage*

Definitions

Recurrent miscarriage describes 3 or more consecutive pregnancy losses. This obstetric problem affects 1% of all women.

Risk factors

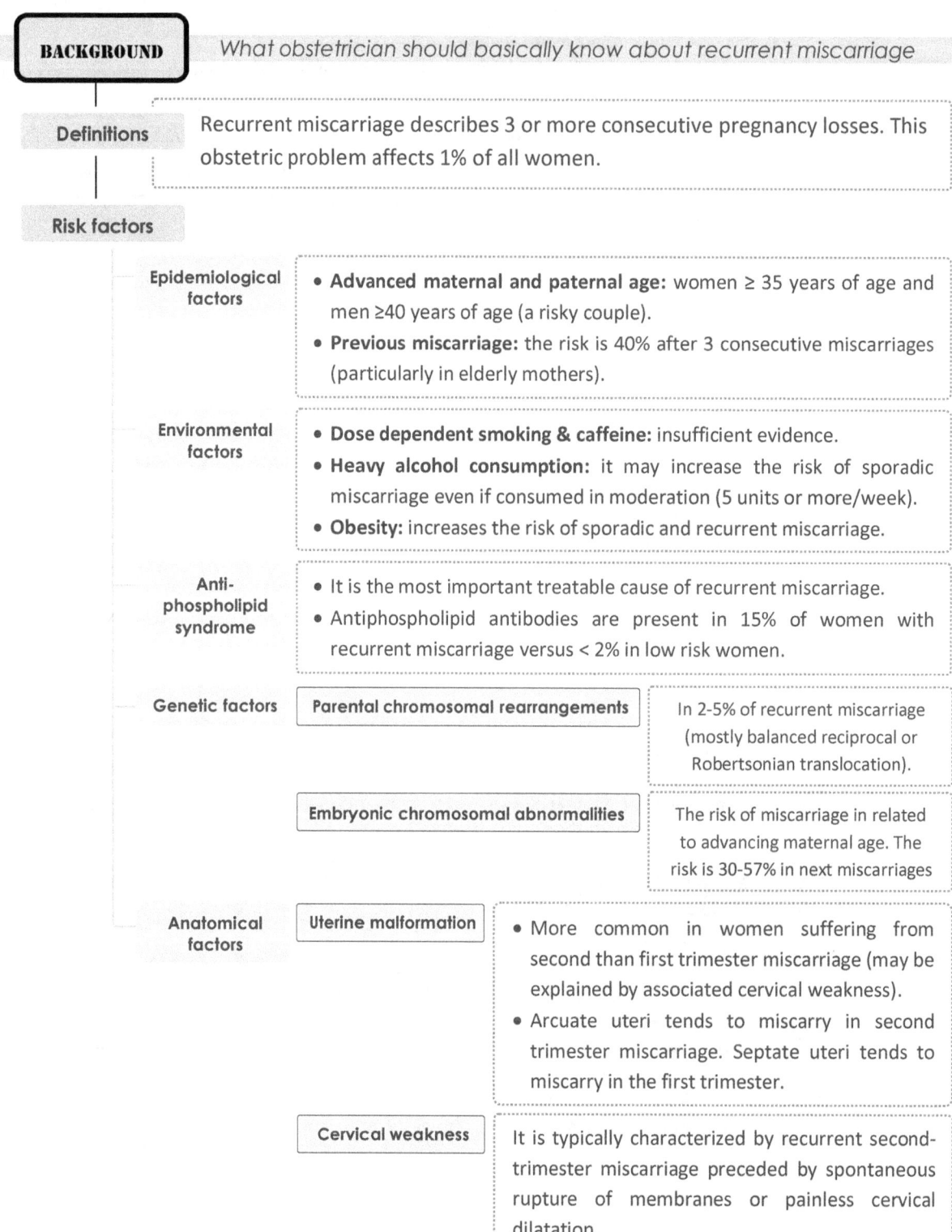

Epidemiological factors
- **Advanced maternal and paternal age:** women ≥ 35 years of age and men ≥40 years of age (a risky couple).
- **Previous miscarriage:** the risk is 40% after 3 consecutive miscarriages (particularly in elderly mothers).

Environmental factors
- **Dose dependent smoking & caffeine:** insufficient evidence.
- **Heavy alcohol consumption:** it may increase the risk of sporadic miscarriage even if consumed in moderation (5 units or more/week).
- **Obesity:** increases the risk of sporadic and recurrent miscarriage.

Anti-phospholipid syndrome
- It is the most important treatable cause of recurrent miscarriage.
- Antiphospholipid antibodies are present in 15% of women with recurrent miscarriage versus < 2% in low risk women.

Genetic factors

| Parental chromosomal rearrangements | In 2-5% of recurrent miscarriage (mostly balanced reciprocal or Robertsonian translocation). |

| Embryonic chromosomal abnormalities | The risk of miscarriage in related to advancing maternal age. The risk is 30-57% in next miscarriages |

Anatomical factors

| Uterine malformation | - More common in women suffering from second than first trimester miscarriage (may be explained by associated cervical weakness).
- Arcuate uteri tends to miscarry in second trimester miscarriage. Septate uteri tends to miscarry in the first trimester. |

| Cervical weakness | It is typically characterized by recurrent second-trimester miscarriage preceded by spontaneous rupture of membranes or painless cervical dilatation. |

Risk factors (cont.)

Endocrine factors	Diabetes mellitus	• Uncontrolled diabetes (indicated by high HB A1c) are at risk of first trimester miscarriage. • Controlled diabetes is not a risk factor.
	Thyroid dysfunction	• Anti-thyroid antibodies are possible cause of recurrent miscarriage. • Treated thyroid dysfunction is not a risk factor
	Polycystic ovary syndrome	• Insulin resistance, hyperinsulinaemia and hyperandrogenaemia explain the risk. • An elevated free androgen index predicts for risk of subsequent miscarriage in women with recurrent miscarriage.
Immune factors	HLA incompatibility	HLA incompatibility between couples, absence of maternal leucocytotoxic antibodies or maternal blocking antibodies should not be investigated routinely. There is no evidence to support a causal relationship between these factors and recurrent miscarriage.
	Natural killer cells	Uterine natural killer (uNK) cells differ in function and shape from peripheral natural killer (NK) cells. Altered peripheral NK cells may be related to recurrent miscarriage. However, this is not supported by evidence and should not be investigated routinely.
	Cytokines	The normal shift to T-helper-2 cell response (which produces anti-inflammatory cytokines e.g. IL 4, 6, 10) over T-helper-1 cell response (produces inflammatory cytokines e.g. IL2, IFN γ, TNF α) occurs during pregnancy. Shift towards TH-1 response is suspected in recurrent miscarriage (needs further research).
Infective factors		• **TORCH and Listeria:** should not be accused or routinely screened. • **Bacterial vaginosis:** first trimester infection predisposes to second trimester miscarriage/preterm labour. Oral clindamycin in early in the second trimester reduces the risk.
Inherited thrombophilias		They are suggestive causes of recurrent miscarriage and late pregnancy complications (possibly due to thrombosis of uteroplacental circulation).

APPROACH   *How obstetricians should deal with recurrent miscarriage*

	Indications for testing	Assessment	Treatment
Anti-phospholipid syndrome	• All women with recurrent 1st trimester miscarriage. • All women with 1 or more 2nd trimester miscarriage.	Diagnosis is based on 2 positive tests at least 12 weeks apart for lupus anticoagulant or anti-cardiolipin antibodies of IgG and/or IgM in a medium or high titre over 40 ml/l or > the 99th percentile).	Low-dose aspirin plus heparin (to prevent further miscarriage). This is no rule for steroids or immunoglobulin.
Cytogenetic (genetic) analysis	Third and subsequent consecutive miscarriage(s) are indication for genetic analysis. This provides data about the prognosis.	Cytogenetic analysis of the products of conception. This may reveal: • **Fetal aneuploidy:** the risk of miscarriage decreases with an increasing number of miscarriages (better prognosis in next the pregnancy). • **Unbalanced structural chromosomal abnormality:** if so, parental peripheral blood karyotyping of both partners is indicated. Abnormalities indicated referral to clinical geneticist to determine prognosis.	Chromosomal rearrangements treatment include: • Proceeding to a further natural pregnancy with or without a prenatal diagnosis test. • Gamete donation. • Adoption. IVF and Preimplantation genetic screening do not improve outcome in unexplained miscarriage
Anatomical factors	All women with recurrent 1st trimester miscarriage and all women with 1 or more 2nd trimester miscarriages	• **Initial screening tests:** 2D pelvic ultrasound and/or HSG. • **Tests for definitive diagnosis:** combined hysteroscopy and laparoscopy ± 3D ultrasound scanning. The rule of MRI is controversial.	• **Congenital uterine malformations:** septum resection value is not supported by sufficient evidence. • **Cervical weakness:** cerclage (see later).
Thrombophilias	Women with second-trimester miscarriage should be screened for inherited thrombophilia	screened for inherited thrombophilias including factor V Leiden, factor II (prothrombin) genemutation and protein S.	Heparin therapy during pregnancy may improve the live birth rate (needs evidence).
Endocrine factors	All women with recurrent miscarriage (particularly 1st trimester)	Testing for diabetes, thyroid function test, polycystic ovary syndrome	Progesterone, HCG, LH suppression (in PCOS patients), metformin are not supported by sufficient evidence
Immune factors	These should not be routinely investigated or treated (only for research). Paternal cell immunisation, 3rd party donor leucocytes, trophoblast membranes and IV immunoglobulin have no rule in unexplained recurrent miscarriage.		
Unexplained	Unexplained recurrent miscarriage has an excellent prognosis for future pregnancy without treatment. Only supportive care in early pregnancy assessment unit is needed.		

Fact Box: Anti-phospholipid syndrome

- Antiphospholipid antibody syndrome is related to anti-phospholipid antibodies (lupus anticoagulant, anticardiolipin antibodies and anti-B2 glycoprotein-I antibodies).
- **For assessment of Antiphospholipid syndrome:** lupus anticoagulant, anticardiolipin antibodies are assessed by:
  - *For lupus anticoagulant:* the dilute Russell's viper venom time test and platelet neutralisation procedure are more sensitive and specific than activated partial thromboplastin time test or the kaolin clotting time test.
  - *For anticardiolipin antibodies:* detected using a standardised ELISA.
- **Percussions and problems:**
  - Temporal fluctuation of antibody titres in individual women.
  - Transient positivity with infections.
  - Suboptimal sample collection and preparation and lack of standardization of laboratory tests can influence the results.

History induced cerclage

Definition

Insertion of a cerclage based on woman's obstetric or gynaecological history.

Indications

- 3 or more previous preterm births and/or second-trimester losses.
- Suggestive features (e.g. painless dilatation of the cervix or rupture of the membranes before the onset of contractions) or history of cervical surgery are not evident to indicate cerclage.
- The use of prepregnancy diagnostic techniques for cervical weakness in suspected women (e.g. Cervical resistance index *, hysterography or insertion of cervical dilators) is not evident as an indication of history induced cerclage.

Timing

A history-indicated suture is performed as prophylaxis in asymptomatic women at 12–14 weeks of gestation.

Ultrasound induced cerclage

Definition

Insertion of a cerclage based on cervical length shortening as diagnosed by transvaginal ultrasound.

Indications

- Women with a history of 1 or more spontaneous mid-trimester losses or preterm births should be followed with transvaginal Sonography of cervical length. Cerclage is indicated if the cervix is 25 mm or less and before 24 weeks of gestation. There is no indication if there is cervical funneling without shortening or shortening without history of spontaneous pregnancy loss or preterm labour.
- Women candidate for a history-indicated cerclage who have undergone the procedure can be followed up by sonographic surveillance for cervical shortening.

Timing

Whenever the cervix is shortened while the cervix is followed up between 14 and 24 weeks of gestation.

Cervical cerclage (based on indication)

Rescue cerclage

Definition

Insertion of cerclage as a salvage for premature cervical dilatation with exposed fetal membranes in the vagina.

Indications

A senior obstetrician-based decision is made for women with premature cervical dilatation and exposed fetal membranes in the vagina (diagnosed clinically or by ultrasound in response to specific complains e.g. vaginal bleeding, discharge, heaviness). The decision depends on 2 arms:
- The advantage of delaying labour for ± 5 weeks with 2 fold reduction in delivery > 34 weeks
- The high risk of severe preterm delivery and neonatal mortality and morbidity even with cerclage. There is also high failure rate of cerclage with > 4 cm cervical dilation and membrane prolapse beyond the external os.

Timing

No evidence of superiority of immediate versus delayed procedure in either rescue or ultrasound indicated cerclage (however, delayed procedure may increase the risk of infection).

* Cervical resistance index: force required to dilate the cervix to 8 mm

** Expectant management may be used as an alternative to serial ultrasounds. Women with a history of second-trimester loss/preterm delivery mostly deliver after 33 weeks of gestation

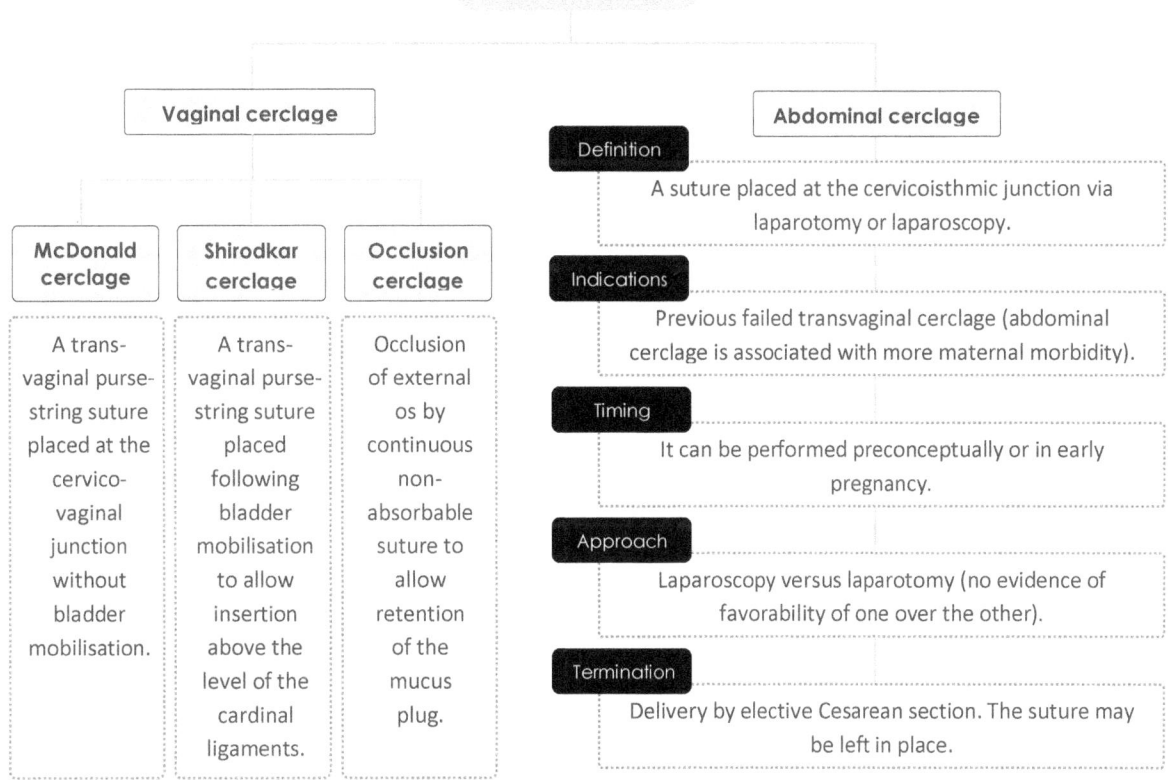

Cervical cerclage (based on approach)

Vaginal cerclage

McDonald cerclage
A transvaginal purse-string suture placed at the cervico-vaginal junction without bladder mobilisation.

Shirodkar cerclage
A transvaginal purse-string suture placed following bladder mobilisation to allow insertion above the level of the cardinal ligaments.

Occlusion cerclage
Occlusion of external os by continuous non-absorbable suture to allow retention of the mucus plug.

Abdominal cerclage

Definition
A suture placed at the cervicoisthmic junction via laparotomy or laparoscopy.

Indications
Previous failed transvaginal cerclage (abdominal cerclage is associated with more maternal morbidity).

Timing
It can be performed preconceptually or in early pregnancy.

Approach
Laparoscopy versus laparotomy (no evidence of favorability of one over the other).

Termination
Delivery by elective Cesarean section. The suture may be left in place.

Fact Box: Special situations with abdominal cerclage

Delayed miscarriage or fetal death in women with an abdominal cerclage is a challenging situation that needs a senior obstetrician with adequate skill in this procedure to take a decision. Options include:

- Suction curettage or dilatation and evacuation (up to 18 weeks of gestation) through the stitch.
- Cutting the suture via a posterior colpotomy.
- Hysterotomy or caesarean section if other measures fail.

Management of cerclage

Cerclage does not cause

Increased risk of PPROM, induction of labour, caesarean section, preterm delivery or second trimester loss

Cerclage may cause

Pyrexia (not chorioamnionitis). Intraoperative bladder damage (small risk), cervical trauma, membrane rupture and bleeding. Risk of anaesthesia during removal of Shirodkar cerclage. Cervical laceration/trauma if labour starts with the suture in place.

Not a routine, only before rescue or ultrasound indicated cerclage when there is intrauterine infection (1-2%) **Inform the woman that it does not increase the risk of preterm delivery before 28 weeks.**

Proper selection of women

Clear indication of cerclage based on history, serial ultrasound or clinical presentation (as mentioned)

Exclusion criteria

> Active preterm labour
> Clinical evidence of chorioamnionitis
> Continuing vaginal bleeding
> PPROM
> Fetal compromise
> Lethal fetal defect
> Fetal death.

Preoperative counseling

Information about possible complications of cerclage

Preoperative assessment

Ultrasound screen

Amniocentesis

Screening for genital infection

Screening for viability, exclusion of aneuploidy & major fetal anomalies

Only if suspicious, positive culture of vaginal swab indicates complete antibiotic course before suturing. **No data supports genital tract infection as a routine**

Preoperative treatment

There is no evidence to support peri-operative tocolytics or antibiotics

There is no evidence to support two purse-string sutures over a single suture or to support cervical occlusion suture in addition to the primary cerclage.

The choice of suture material and technique (McDonald versus Shirodkar) is the discretion of the team.

Anaesthesia

General versus regional anaesthesia (no evidence of difference, it is the discretion of the team)

The procedure

Transvaginal cerclage

A day case procedure

Rescue/ultrasound cerclage

At least 24 hour hospital observation

Abdominal cerclage

At least 48 hours

Postoperative care

Hospital stay

Bed rest	Intercourse	Progesterone	Fetal fibronectin	Serial ultrasound
Not a routine, indicated on individual basis	Abstinence is not routinely recommended	Routine use is not indicated as a supplement	Not a routine, high negative predictive value provides reassurance in certain cases. Positive results are less valued (high false positive results)	May be valuable in US-indicated cerclage (for timely administration of steroids). Upper cervical length < 10 mm before 28 weeks indicates preterm labour < 36 weeks

Transvaginal cerclage is removed at 36-37 weeks, at elective Cesarean section or if preterm labour is established

Cerclage removal

Abdominal cerclage is left in place. This is not known to cause long-term problems and is reasonable if further pregnancies are expected

Fact Box: Management of cervical cerclage

- Preoperative WBC and C-reactive protein before rescue cerclage (to diagnose infection) are not recommended unless clinically indicated.
- The value of amnioreduction before rescue cerclage is controversial.
- Postoperative upper cervical length (closed cervix above cerclage) is detected by transvaginal ultrasound following ultrasound indicated cerclage.

Appendix   **Cerclage in certain obstetric situations**

Multiple pregnancy

The insertion of a history- or ultrasound-indicated cerclage in women with multiple pregnancies is not recommended because it may be associated with an increase in preterm delivery and pregnancy loss.

Uterine anomalies

History- or ultrasound-indicated cerclage is not recommended in women with müllerian anomalies.

Cervical trauma

History- or ultrasound-indicated cerclage is not recommended in women with previous cervical surgery (cone biopsy, large loop excision of the transformation zone or destructive procedures (laser ablation or diathermy) or multiple dilatation and evacuation.

The decision to place a cerclage in women who had **radical trachelectomy** should be individualized.

PPROM

- **In women with PPROM between 24 and 34 weeks of gestation:** if there is no evidence of infection or preterm labour, delayed removal of the cerclage (for 48 hours) may be beneficial for a course of prophylactic steroids to be completed and/or in utero transfer to be arranged.
  However, delayed suture removal until labour or until delivery is indicated not recommended because it is associated with an increased risk of maternal/fetal sepsis
- **In women with PPROM before 23 and after 34 weeks of gestation:** the risk of neonatal and/or maternal sepsis is considerable and the benefit of 48 hours of latency is minimal. Immediate removal of the cerclage is recommended.

Post-cerclage cervical shortening

- An ultrasound-indicated cerclage due to cervical length shortening is not recommended over expectant management because this may be associated with an increase in both pregnancy loss and delivery before 35 weeks of gestation.
- A rescue cerclage following history or ultrasound-indicated cerclage is an individualized decision according to circumstances.

STATION 3: EARLY OBSTETRIC COMPLICATIONS

Ectopic pregnancy

BACKGROUND — *What obstetrician should basically know about ectopic pregnancy*

Definitions

Ectopic pregnancy is an abnormal pregnancy that implants outside the uterine cavity.

Incidence

- The incidence in UK is 11.1 per 1000 pregnancies.
- It accounts for about 7.5% of all direct maternal deaths (10 maternal deaths in 2003 – 2005). However, maternal mortality has decreased about 4 fold in the last 20 years as a result of early detection and proper management protocols.

Types

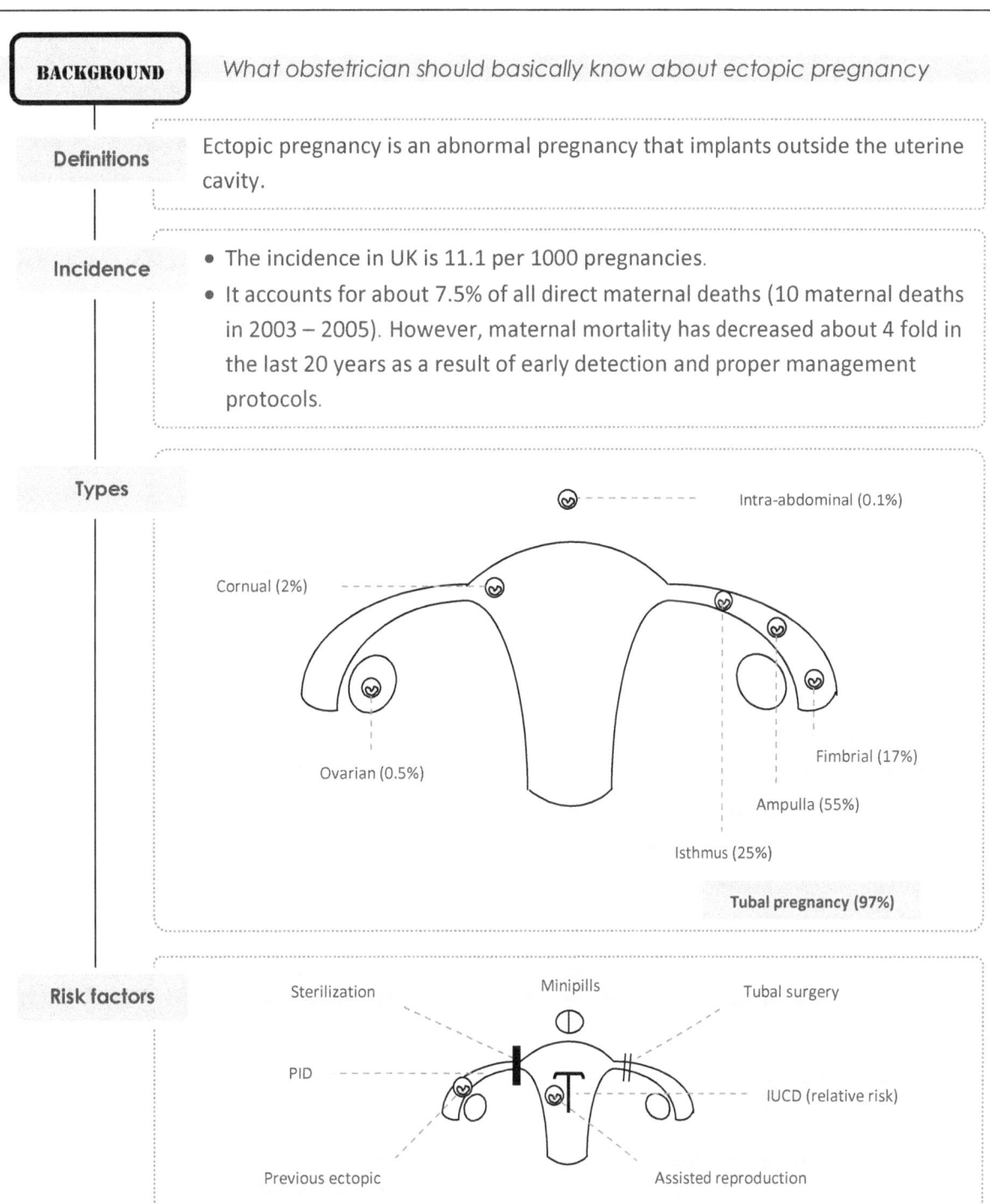

Intra-abdominal (0.1%)

Cornual (2%)

Ovarian (0.5%)

Fimbrial (17%)

Ampulla (55%)

Isthmus (25%)

Tubal pregnancy (97%)

Risk factors

Sterilization — Minipills — Tubal surgery

PID

IUCD (relative risk)

Previous ectopic — Assisted reproduction

* All contraceptives provide a lower risk of ectopic pregnancy than if no contraception is used. However, the risk of ectopic pregnancy is 3 times higher in IUCD users than with other contraceptives (relative risk).

** Depot medroxyprogesterone acetate provides a lower risk of ectopic pregnancy than the mini-pill but higher than the COCP.

APPROACH   *How obstetricians should deal with ectopic pregnancy*

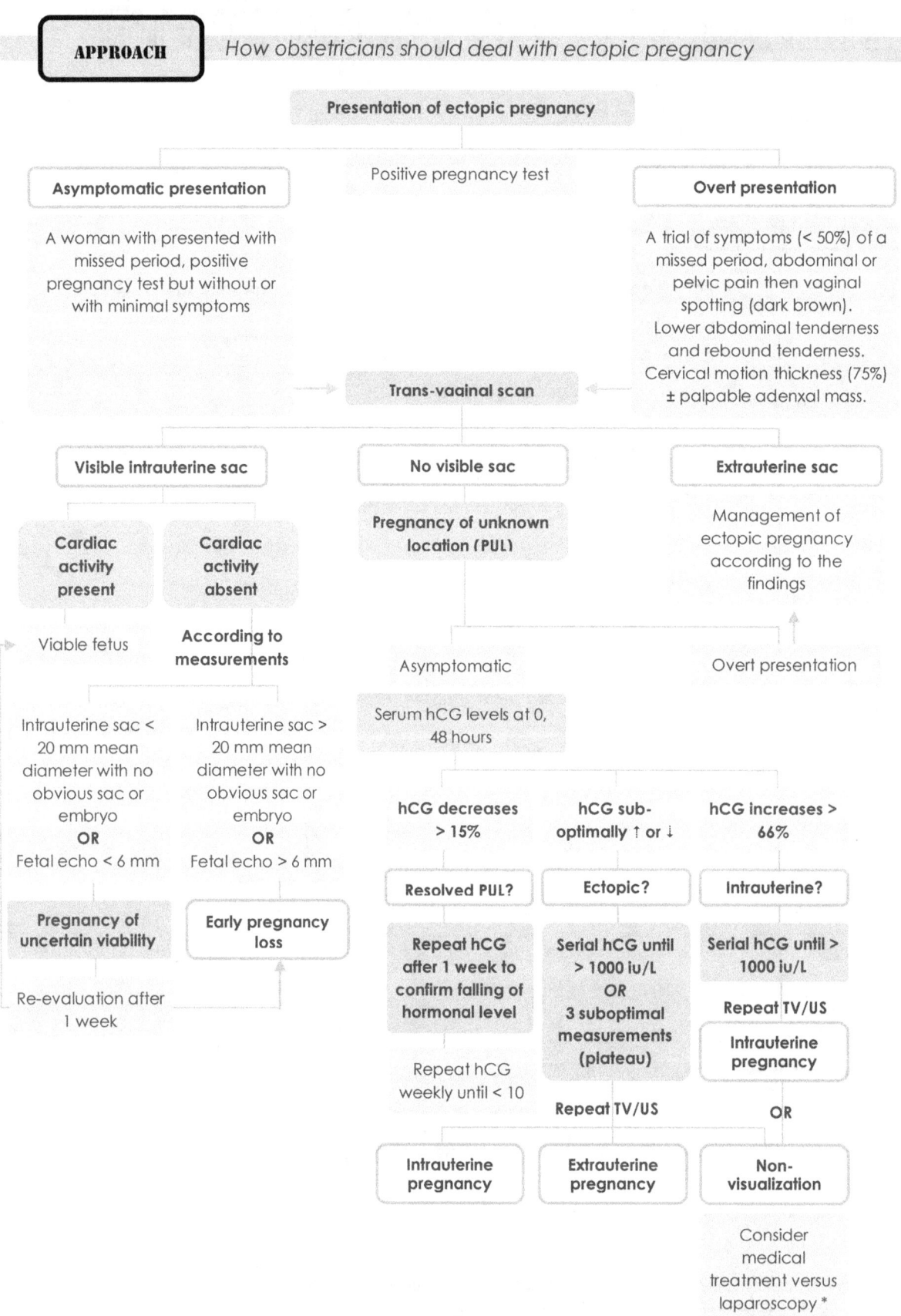

Presentation of ectopic pregnancy

Asymptomatic presentation

Positive pregnancy test

Overt presentation

A woman with presented with missed period, positive pregnancy test but without or with minimal symptoms

A trial of symptoms (< 50%) of a missed period, abdominal or pelvic pain then vaginal spotting (dark brown). Lower abdominal tenderness and rebound tenderness. Cervical motion thickness (75%) ± palpable adenxal mass.

Trans-vaginal scan

Visible intrauterine sac

No visible sac

Extrauterine sac

Pregnancy of unknown location (PUL)

Management of ectopic pregnancy according to the findings

Cardiac activity present

Cardiac activity absent

Viable fetus

According to measurements

Asymptomatic

Overt presentation

Intrauterine sac < 20 mm mean diameter with no obvious sac or embryo
OR
Fetal echo < 6 mm

Intrauterine sac > 20 mm mean diameter with no obvious sac or embryo
OR
Fetal echo > 6 mm

Serum hCG levels at 0, 48 hours

Pregnancy of uncertain viability

Early pregnancy loss

Re-evaluation after 1 week

hCG decreases > 15%

hCG sub-optimally ↑ or ↓

hCG increases > 66%

Resolved PUL?

Ectopic?

Intrauterine?

Repeat hCG after 1 week to confirm falling of hormonal level

Serial hCG until > 1000 iu/L
OR
3 suboptimal measurements (plateau)

Serial hCG until > 1000 iu/L

Repeat TV/US

Repeat hCG weekly until < 10

Repeat TV/US

Intrauterine pregnancy

OR

Intrauterine pregnancy

Extrauterine pregnancy

Non-visualization

Consider medical treatment versus laparoscopy *

* Diagnostic laparoscopy has a false positive rate of 5% and a false negative rate of 3-4%.

A woman with ectopic pregnancy

Haemodynamically stable

Clinical, sonographic and laboratory assessment of the patient

IF

Haemodynamically instable

Resuscitation and immediate laparotomy (complete/partial salpingectomy)

- Woman is counseled and is able to comply with close follow-up
- No fetal cardiac activity in ectopic mass
- Initial HCG < 3000 iu/l

- An asymptomatic and haemodynamically stable woman.
- HCG low and falling (<1000 iu/l).
- < 100ml blood in pouch of Douglas.
- No cardiac activity in ectopic mass.
- Low and rapidly falling HCG levels (initial fall > 15% at 0, 48 hour hCG).
- Woman's acceptance supported by written information

- If the criteria of medical or expectant management are not met.
- If these options are not accepted by the woman

Medical treatment

Intra-muscular methotrexate – 50 mg/m² body surface area

Follow up

Serum ß-hCG is measured on days 4 and 7. If hCG falls by < 15% between days 4 and 7, a further dose of methotrexate is given.

Expectant treatment

Perform twice weekly serum hCG and weekly transvaginal scans to confirm a rapid falling hCG level and a decrease in the size of ectopic mass.
Then, weekly HCG and scans are performed until HCG is <20 iu/l.

Surgical treatment

- If pelvic adhesions are present.
- If hematoperitoneum is identified.
- If pregnancy is > 4 cm,
- If the woman becomes hemodynamic instable.

Laparoscopy versus laparotomy

YES

NO

Laparotomy

Laparoscopy

If the other tube is unhealthy or

If the other tube is intact and healthy

Salpingectomy

Salpingostomy

Tubal conservation should be considered (subsequent intrauterine pregnancy rate is 54% versus 20.5% risk of recurrence)

Salpingotomy vs. salpingectomy Subsequent intra-uterine pregnancy rate is 46 vs. 44%. More recurrence and risk of persistent trophoblastic disease after salpinotomy

- If the tube continues to bleed after Salpingostomy.
- If the tube is unhealthy or pregnancy is recurrent at the same tube

Conservative surgery is the classic procedure by laparoscopy

Follow up hCG weekly

Medical treatment: How to counsel your patient?

Approach

- Women should be able to comply with treatment and follow-up.
- Treatment consists of a single injection of IM methotrexate (50 mg/m^2). Beta-HCG is followed up on days 4 and 7 (not before day 4 because a transient increase in beta-HCG may occur in up to 86% of women between days 1 and 4 of treatment).
- Serum beta-HCG is expected to decrease > 15% between days 4 and 7. A further dose of methotrexate should be considered if this decrease is not achieved (14% of women require more than one dose).
- Before treatment is given, a woman should be informed that she may experience the following during treatment:
  - Abdominal pain in 75% of women, increase in abdominal pain in 59% of women after methotrexate is given.
  - Tubal rupture during follow-up in 7% of women. So, women should be informed (with written information) that they may need further treatment and its potential complications (<10% require surgical intervention).
  - Subsequent intra-uterine pregnancy rate is 54% and recurrent ectopic rates are 8-10%.

Advantages

- Success rates of 85-94% following single dose treatment.
- Less expensive.
- Fewer side-effects.
- It requires less intensive monitoring and does not require folinic acid adjuvant (versus multiple dose regimens).

Disadvantages

The following complications may develop: Stomatitis, alopecia, haematosalpinx, neutropaenia, pneumonitis, multiple ovarian cysts, failed therapy.

Instructions

- Women should be advised to avoid sexual intercourse during treatment.
- Women should maintain ample fluid intake during treatment.
- Women should use an effective contraception for 3 months after treatment because methotrexate is teratogenic.

Expectant treatment: How to counsel your patient?

- Provide clear written information about this management including the importance of compliance with follow-up.
- Easy access to the hospital should be ensured.
- Woman should be informed that intervention may be required in 23-29% of cases. Tubal rupture may occur even during the rapid falling of hCG.

Surgical treatment: How to counsel your patient?

Laparotomy vs. laparoscopy

Whenever the patient is haemodynamically stable, laparoscopy is preferable over laparotomy.

Advantages of laparoscopy over laparotomy

- Lower blood loss
- Lower analgesic requirement
- Shorter hospital stay
- Quicker post-operative recovery
- Lower cost
- Possibly lower repeat ectopic pregnancy rate
- Lower risk of adhesion formation
- No significant difference in subsequent intra-uterine pregnancy rates

Disadvantages of laparoscopy compared to laparotomy

- Higher rate of persistent trophoblastic tissue (12.2% v 1.7%) if salpingotomy performed

Salpingectomy vs. salpingotomy

The choice of the surgical procedure depends on clinical circumstances. However, the surgeon and the patient should be aware of these points

Subsequent intrauterine pregnancy rate	• *If the other tube is present and is apparently healthy:* subsequent intra-uterine pregnancy rate does not differ significantly (46 vs. 44%). • *If the other tube is diseased or absent:* tubal conservation associated with a 54% intra-uterine pregnancy rate but a 20.5% recurrent ectopic pregnancy rate. Counseling about the need and cost of IVF should be considered preoperatively.
Postoperative complications	Risk of tubal bleeding in the immediate post-op period and persistent trophoblastic tissue are higher after Salpingotomy. This should be discussed and documented.
Recurrence	Recurrent ectopic pregnancy rate appears to be higher after Salpingotomy. However, available data is still conflicting.

Consent form for laparoscopic management of tubal ectopic pregnancy

The name of the procedure	Laparoscopic salpingectomy or salpingotomy. This is the procedure to be performed after confirmation of ectopic pregnancy.
The principle of the procedure	Give information about the nature of laparoscopy, salpingectomy or salpingotomy. Any additional procedure should be discussed with the woman (laparotomy, salpingectomy, repair of damage to bowel, bladder, uterus or blood vessels, blood transfusion and oophorectomy).
The expected benefit	The procedure confirms the diagnosis and remove the ectopic pregnancy. There will be less blood loss, hospital stay and quicker recovery (see before).
The possible risks	
Serious risks	• Bowel, bladder, uterine injury or major blood vessel injury. She should be informed that these complications are rare (2:1000) but requires immediate repair by laparoscopy or laparotomy (uncommon). However, Up to 15% of bowel injuries are undiscovered at the time of laparoscopy. • Failure of the procedure is possible (either to gain entry or to complete the procedure efficiently). The woman should be informed that this requires laparotomy. • The risk of death as a result of complications is extremely low (3-4:100 000).
Frequent risks	Woman should be informed that some minor but frequent problems may develop during the procedure. This includes: inability to identify the diagnosis, bruising, shoulder-tip pain, wound gaping or infection, hernia at site of entry, persistent trophoblastic tissue (only Salpingotomy, 4–8%).
Alternative treatments	Other treatment options including laparotomy, medical treatment and expectant management should be discussed.
Statement of the patient	Procedures that are appropriate (but not essential) should be discussed. The woman's wishes should be reported after counseling.
Anaesthesia and obesity	The route of anaesthesia should be discussed with the woman in details. The risk of obesity (both surgical and anesthetic risk) should be explained.

Written information should always support your discussion.

STATION 3: EARLY OBSTETRIC COMPLICATIONS

Vomiting with pregnancy

BACKGROUND — *What obstetrician should know about vomiting with pregnancy*

Definitions

- Nausea and vomiting are common during early pregnancy. However, hyperemesis gravidarum is a term that describes the extreme degree of vomiting in early pregnancy that is based mainly on patient's perception of severity rather than on certain clinical classification.
- Hyperemesis gravidarum is vomiting related to early pregnancy which is severe enough to affect the general condition of the woman and to require hospital admission.
- Hyperemesis gravidarum is a clinical diagnosis of exclusion which meets the following criteria:
  - Persistent severe vomiting not explained by other causes.
  - Acute starvation (large ketonuria).
  - At least 3% weight loss of the pre-pregnancy weight.
  - ± Electrolyte, liver or thyroid dysfunction.

Incidence

- 50% of pregnant women experience nausea and vomiting. 25% experience nausea only and 25% do not suffer.
- Hyperemesis gravidarum affects only 3-10 women per 1000 pregnancies. The peak incidence is between 8 and 12 weeks and is unusual after 16 weeks gestation
- Recurrence rate is about 50%.

Risk factors

- Increased placental mass (e.g. molar gestation, multiple gestation).
- Family history (genetic factor).
- History of hyperemesis gravidarum in a previous pregnancy.
- History of motion sickness or migraine.

Complications

Maternal complications

- Wernicke's encephalopathy (vitamin B1 deficiency).
- Splenic avulsion, Mallory-Weiss tears and esophageal rupture.
- Pneumothorax.
- Acute tubular necrosis and liver dysfunction (jaundice).
- Psychosocial morbidity including depression, somatization, and hypochondriasis.
- Dehydration, malnutrition and electrolyte imbalance. Venous thromboembolism.

Fetal complications

- Mild and moderate vomiting is not associated with adverse fetal outcome. Severe vomiting may be associated with low birth weight (LBW).
- Some cases of fetal death are reported with extreme hyperemesis gravidarum

APPROACH   *How obstetricians should deal with vomiting with pregnancy*

Vomiting with pregnancy

History

| Exclusion of other diagnoses | | Assessment of severity |

GIT symptoms (diarrhea, constipation, pain)   Assessment by scoring systems e.g. frequency *

GUT symptoms (loin pain, frequency, dysuria)   Assessment by impaction on the quality of life

Examination

| General examination | | Local examination |

Assessment of dehydration including mucous membranes, skin turgor, pulse and blood pressure – Assessment of jaundice

Assessment of the abdomen and the pelvis e.g. loin, regional abdominal tenderness or masses

Investigations

Blood tests		Serum electrolytes
Liver function and enzymes		Serum amylase
Thyroid function		Urine analysis

TSH is slightly depressed in the first trimester

For leucocytes, protein, nitrites, and ketones

Exclusion of other causes based on these data

CNS	GIT	GUT	Metabolic	Obstetric
• Tumors of the central nervous system • Pseudotumor cerebri • Vestibular lesions • Migraine • Psychologic disorders	• Achalasia • Peptic ulcer • Pancreatitis • Hepatitis • Biliary tract disease • Intestinal obstruction • Gastroenteritis • Gastroparesis • Appendicitis	• Pyelonephritis • Renal failure • Kidney stones • Ovarian torsion • Degenerating leiomyoma	• Diabetic ketoacidosis • Porphyria • Addison's disease • Hyperthyroidism • Drug toxicity or intolerance	• Acute fatty liver of pregnancy • Preeclampsia

| Pelvic Ultrasound |

Exclude multiple pregnancy, molar pregnancy

Final diagnosis of emesis gravidarum by exclusion
Final diagnosis of hyperemesis by affection of the general condition and development of complications

* Scoring systems may depend on the frequency or the duration of vomiting. However, their clinical impact is questionable.

Vomiting with pregnancy

Mild/moderate vomiting *

Diet modification

- Avoid spicy food.
- Eat small regular meals
- Avoid drugs that disturb the GI tract e.g. iron preparations

Non-pharmacological

Non-pharmacological options may be tried prior to drug therapy:
- Ginger cap (250mg X4)
- P6 acupuncture

No response

Pharmacological treatment

Vitamin B6 10–25 mg, 3 or 4 times per day (up to 40 mg)

If no response, Add:

Doxylamine 12.5 mg, 3 or 4 times per day

If no response, Add:

Promethazine 12.5–25 mg every 4 hours, orally or rectally

Dimenhydrinate 50–100 mg every 4–6 hours, orally or rectally

If no response

Severe vomiting **

No dehydration

Metoclopramide, 5–10 mg every 8 hours intramuscularly

OR

Promethazine 12.5–25 mg every 4 hours intramuscularly or rectally

OR

Trimethobenzamide, 200 mg every 6-8 hours, rectally

Dehydration***

IV fluid therapy (avoid dextrose)

Plus

Dimenhydrinate 50 mg (in 50 mL saline, over 20 min) IV every 4–6 hours

OR

Metoclopramide, 5–10 mg every 8 hours, intravenously

OR

Promethazine, 12.5–25 mg every 4 hours, intravenously

If no response, Add:

Methylprednisolone 16 mg every 8 hours IV or oral, for 3 days. Taper over 2 weeks to lowest effective dose.

OR

Ondansetron 8 mg, over 15 minutes, every 12 hours, intravenously

Consider thiamine therapy to prevent Wernike's encephalopathy

---

* Reassurance and emotional support is indicated. The therapeutic rule of psychotherapy is still questionable. She should be informed that it will mostly resolve spontaneously by 16 - 20 weeks and is not usually associated with poor pregnancy outcomes

Early treatment is thought to reduce the risk of progression into severe vomiting.

** Hospitalization is recommended in severe cases when oral fluids cannot be tolerated. Exclusion of other causes and IV treatment are indicated. Follow up during treatment is indicated:

- Assessment of pulse and blood pressure every 4-6 hours.
- Fluid balance chart
- Daily urine dipstix for ketones
- Weigh the patient twice weekly

Patient is counseled for termination of pregnancy only in very severe cases refractory to all treatment lines.

*** Dehydration along with immobilization and pregnancy may increase the risk of venous thromboembolism

Thromboprophylaxis is indicated.

CHAPTER 4
THE ANTEPARTUM PERIOD

STATION 4: LATE OBSTETRIC HAEMORRHAGE

Antepartum haemorrhage

BACKGROUND   *What obstetrician should know about Antepartum haemorrhage*

Definitions

Bleeding from or into the genital tract after the gestation age for fetal viability (24 weeks).

Incidence

- Antepartum haemorrhage (APH) complicates 3-5% of pregnancies.
- APH is responsible for 20% of very preterm deliveries.

Causes

- Placenta previa (30%) which is a placenta that is implanted wholly or partially in the lower uterine segment.
  The overall incidence is 28% before 24 weeks of gestation, 3% at term.
- Placental abruption (20%) which is bleeding from premature separation of a normally cited placenta.
  The overall incidence is 0.5 - 1.8% (20-35% of cases are concealed).
- Vasa previa.
- Incidental bleeding from local genital causes e.g. genital trauma, cervical polyp or ectropion, labour show, vulvo-vaginal varices or genital tract malignancy and infection.

Risk factors of placenta previa

- Previous placenta praevia (4-8 times).
- Previous caesarean sections:
  - One previous caesarean section OR 2.2.
  - Two previous caesarean sections OR 4.1.
  - Three previous caesarean sections OR 22.4.
- Previous termination of pregnancy
- Multiparity
- Advanced maternal age (>40 years)
- Multiple pregnancy
- Smoking
- Deficient endometrium due to presence or history of:
  - uterine scar
  - endometritis
  - manual removal of placenta
  - curettage
  - submucous fibroid
- Assisted conception

Risk factors of placental abruption

- Previous abruption:
  - 4.4% for one previous abruption.
  - 19–25% for two previous abruption events.
- Pre-eclampsia, fetal growth restriction.
- Non-vertex presentations.
- Polyhydramnios.
- Advanced maternal age.
- Multiparity.
- Low body mass index (BMI).
- Pregnancy following assisted reproductive techniques.
- Intrauterine infection.
- Premature rupture of membranes.
- Abdominal trauma (both accidental and resulting from domestic violence).
- Smoking and drug misuse (cocaine, amphetamines) during pregnancy.
- First trimester bleeding and intrauterine haematoma.
- Maternal thrombophilias (heterozygous factor V Leiden and heterozygous prothrombin 20210A?).

Classification

Placenta previa

- **Placenta pravia major:** if the placenta lies over the internal cervical os.
- **Placenta pravia minor:** if the lower edge of the placenta is in the lower uterine segment but not covering the cervical os.

Placental abruption

- **Grade 0:** Asymptomatic with incidental finding of retro-placental clot.
- **Grade 1:** Vaginal bleeding but no maternal or fetal compromise ± uterine tenderness and irritability.
- **Grade 2:** Fetal distress but NO maternal shock (± vaginal bleeding).
- **Grade 3:** Maternal shock and fetal demise, marked uterine tetany and tenderness (± vaginal bleeding).

Complications

Maternal complications

- Anaemia.
- Maternal shock.
- Complications of blood transfusion.
- Consumptive coagulopathy.
- Postpartum haemorrhage.
- Infection.
- Renal tubular necrosis.
- Psychological complications.
- Prolonged hospital stay.
- Placenta accreta (placenta previa)

Fetal complications

- Prematurity (spontaneous or iatrogenic).
- Small for gestational age and fetal growth restriction.
- Fetal hypoxia.
- Fetal death.

APPROACH *How obstetricians should deal with Antepartum haemorrhage*

First look assessment

No maternal compromise

Compromised clinical state

Immediate resuscitation and stabilization before fetal well-being is assessed

Full clinical assessment

History

R Risk factors of placenta previa, placenta abruption and other causes should be identified.

P Pain. Continuous pain is related to placenta abruption. Intermittent pain is associated with labour. Painless bleeding is related to placenta previa (unless during labour).

R Rupture of membranes. Bleeding related to the onset of bleeding is suggestive of vasa previa.

P Previous cervical smear history may give a clue about cervical pathology.

F Fetal movement. Awareness of fetal movement should be discussed.

Examination

General examination

Pulse, blood pressure, temperature and respiration are reported. Albuminuria is excluded (for pre-eclampsia)*. The ABC approach of airway (A), breathing (B) and circulation (C) is followed.

Ultrasound

Confirmation/exclusion of placenta previa and its degree prior to examination. Retroplacental hematoma is missed in 75% of cases but once diagnosed, it is highly true.

Confirm fetal viability

Abdominal examination

A woody tender uterus on palpation suggests abruption

Soft non-tender uterus suggests placenta, vasa previa or local causes

Palpable intermittent abdominal hardening suggest contractions

Pelvic examination

Placenta previa excluded

Speculum examination

Assess cervical dilation
Assess local genital pathology

Assessment of cervical dilation if there is pain or contractions

Digital examination

Investigations

Maternal investigations

Based on the amount of blood loss

Major bleeding

Complete blood count

Coagulation profile

4 units of blood cross-matched

Kleihauer test to adjust the dose of anti-D serum

Mild bleeding

Full blood count, group and save

If low platelets

Fetal investigations

Fetal tococardiography is indicated after confirmation of fetal viability by ultrasound and whenever fetal condition may influence the decision of management. So it is not indicated if gestation is less than 26 weeks. Abnormal CTG is an indication of delivery in women managed conservatively.

NB

Placental abruption is a clinical diagnosis. Ultrasound and Kleihauer test have a poor diagnostic value in cases of abruption.

* Blood pressure is not conclusive if there is haemorrhagic shock and the diagnosis of preeclampsia may be misleading.

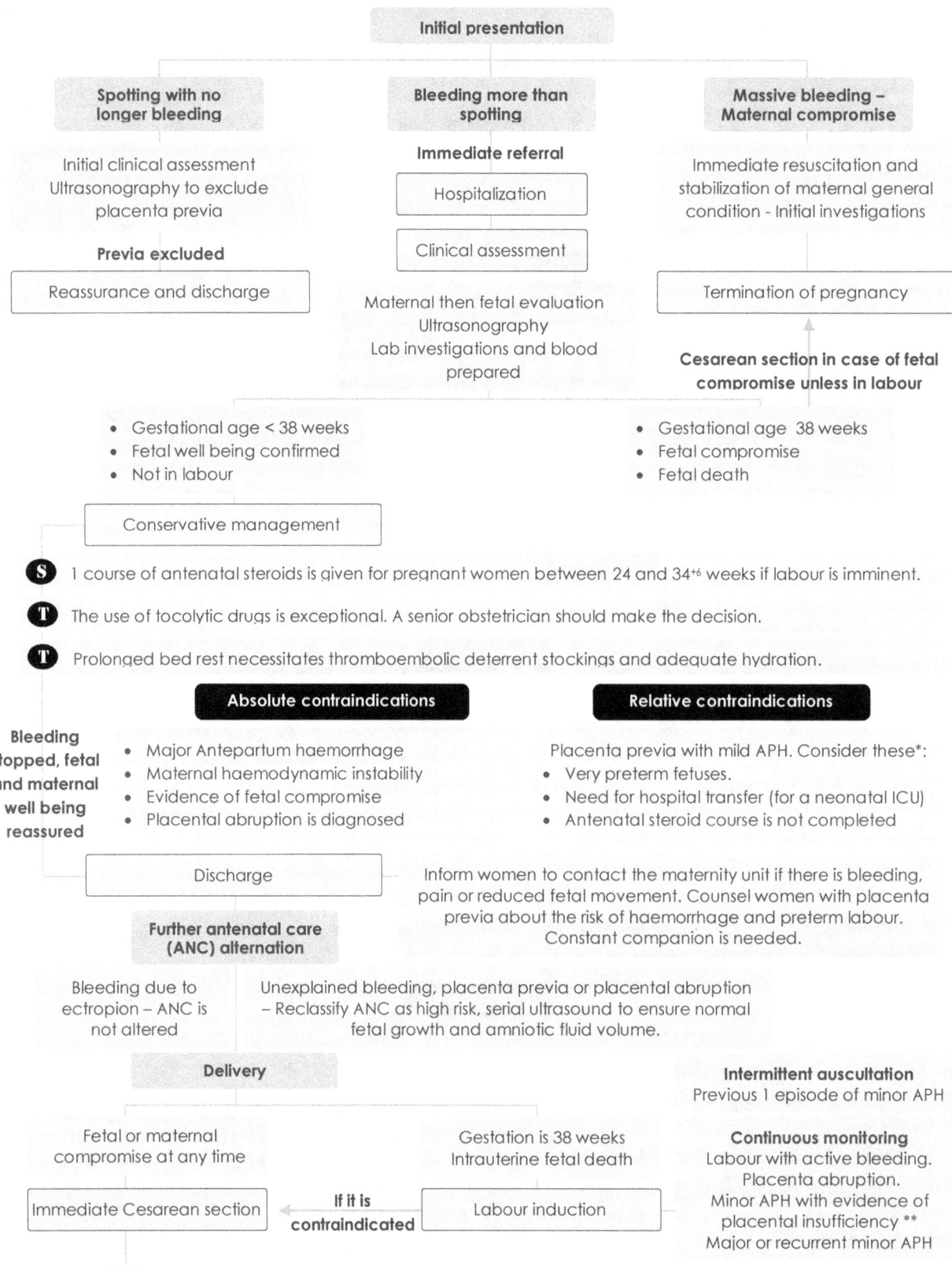

Initial presentation

Spotting with no longer bleeding

Initial clinical assessment
Ultrasonography to exclude placenta previa

Previa excluded

Reassurance and discharge

Bleeding more than spotting

Immediate referral

Hospitalization

Clinical assessment

Maternal then fetal evaluation
Ultrasonography
Lab investigations and blood prepared

Massive bleeding – Maternal compromise

Immediate resuscitation and stabilization of maternal general condition - Initial investigations

Termination of pregnancy

Cesarean section in case of fetal compromise unless in labour

- Gestational age < 38 weeks
- Fetal well being confirmed
- Not in labour

- Gestational age 38 weeks
- Fetal compromise
- Fetal death

Conservative management

S 1 course of antenatal steroids is given for pregnant women between 24 and 34^{+6} weeks if labour is imminent.

T The use of tocolytic drugs is exceptional. A senior obstetrician should make the decision.

T Prolonged bed rest necessitates thromboembolic deterrent stockings and adequate hydration.

Absolute contraindications

Bleeding stopped, fetal and maternal well being reassured

- Major Antepartum haemorrhage
- Maternal haemodynamic instability
- Evidence of fetal compromise
- Placental abruption is diagnosed

Relative contraindications

Placenta previa with mild APH. Consider these*:
- Very preterm fetuses.
- Need for hospital transfer (for a neonatal ICU)
- Antenatal steroid course is not completed

Discharge

Inform women to contact the maternity unit if there is bleeding, pain or reduced fetal movement. Counsel women with placenta previa about the risk of haemorrhage and preterm labour. Constant companion is needed.

Further antenatal care (ANC) alternation

Bleeding due to ectropion – ANC is not altered

Unexplained bleeding, placenta previa or placental abruption – Reclassify ANC as high risk, serial ultrasound to ensure normal fetal growth and amniotic fluid volume.

Delivery

Intermittent auscultation
Previous 1 episode of minor APH

Fetal or maternal compromise at any time

Gestation is 38 weeks
Intrauterine fetal death

Continuous monitoring
Labour with active bleeding.
Placenta abruption.
Minor APH with evidence of placental insufficiency **
Major or recurrent minor APH

Immediate Cesarean section ← **If it is contraindicated**   Labour induction

Consultant anaesthetist attends — Regional anaesthesia is the route unless there is a contraindication (e.g. DIC).

General anaesthesia if there is maternal or fetal compromise

Anaesthetist and maternal decision

* These groups would benefit most from antenatal steroids. Avoid using nifedipine in APH.
** Evidence of placental insufficiency may include fetal growth restriction or oligohydramnios.

Fact Box: Hospitalization and discharge in women with placenta previa

- Symptomatic major placenta previa: should be hospitalized. Bleeding is recurrent and unpredictable. There is no objective judgment to decide discharge.
- Asymptomatic major placenta previa: should be hospitalized during the late third trimester (32-36 weeks). The exact time of admission depends on proximity to hospital, the presence of constant companion and the woman's desire. She should also attend hospital immediately if she develops bleeding, contractions or abdominal pain.

Fact Box: Delivery of women with APH due to placenta previa

- **Mode of delivery (vaginal delivery versus Cesarean section):**
  The mode of delivery is discussed with the woman based on clinical and sonographic data:
  - If the placental edge is < 2 cm from the internal os in the third trimester: Caesarean section is advised especially if the placenta is thick (further research is needed). The thicker the placental edge (over 1 cm), the greater the likelihood of Cesarean section.
  - Trans-vaginal ultrasound scan is acceptable if the fetal head is found engaged prior to a planned Cesarean section. That is because the lower uterine segment continues to grow beyond 36 weeks of gestation.
- **Timing of delivery:**
  Elective delivery is recommended at 38 weeks of gestation to minimize neonatal morbidity. It is not recommended before 38 weeks for placenta previa and 36-37 weeks for suspected placenta accreta.
- **Preoperative preparation:**
  - *Place:* delivery should be carried out in a unit with available blood bank and high dependency care.
  - *Procedures:*
    - *Blood:* cross matched blood available (no need for autologous blood transfusion). Cell salvage is to be considered.
    - *Consent:* prior to delivery, a detailed consent should be taken (see later).
    - *Available critical care:* Local availability of a level 2 critical care bed.
  - *Operative attendance:*
    - A senior experienced obstetrician should be scrubbed in theatre.
    - A consultant obstetrician and anaesthetist should be present in the delivery suite.
    - Consultant staff should be alerted if emergency arises and attends immediately.

Fact Box: Management of massive haemorrhage (careful documentation is essential)

- **Calling for extra-help:** is the first step. There is no place for 'losing face' thinking.
- **Uterotonic agents:** should be considered.
- **Temporary bimanual compression:** or even aortic compression until help is available.
- **Surgical approach:** B-Lynch suture, uterine and internal iliac artery ligation.
- **Interventional radiology:** facilities should be available specially if placenta accreta is suspected and the woman refuses blood transfusion.
  Prophylactic catheter placement for balloon occlusion or in readiness for embolisation needs further evaluation. There may be failure, post-removal bleeding or popliteal arterial thrombus.
- **Hysterectomy:** is the definitive last option

Postpartum management

Management of 3rd stage

- APH is a risk factor for postpartum haemorrhage. Accordingly, the risk should be discussed with the mother including the management of the 3rd stage.
- APH due placenta previa or placental abruption is an indication for active management of the third stage. Whenever there is no hypertension, active management using ergometrine-oxytocin (Syntometrine) is recommended.

Anti-D serum

- A part from routine anti-D serum given to Rh negative mothers, women should be give anti-D serum after any presentation with APH.
- Following an attack of APH (after 20 weeks of gestation), at least 500 iu anti-D Ig is given an then Kleihauer test is performed to estimate feto-maternal haemorrhage > 4 ml to adjust the dose.
- If APH is recurrent, repeat the dose every 6 weeks.

Thromboprophylaxis

- In women with massive APH, immediate thromboprophylaxis should be considered after the risk of haemorrhage subsides. This is because both haemorrhage and blood transfusion are risk factors of thromboembolism.
- If thromboprophylaxis is indicated (high risk) while bleeding is continuous or there is high risk of haemorrhage, unfractionated heparin and/or graduated compression stockings

Neonatal care

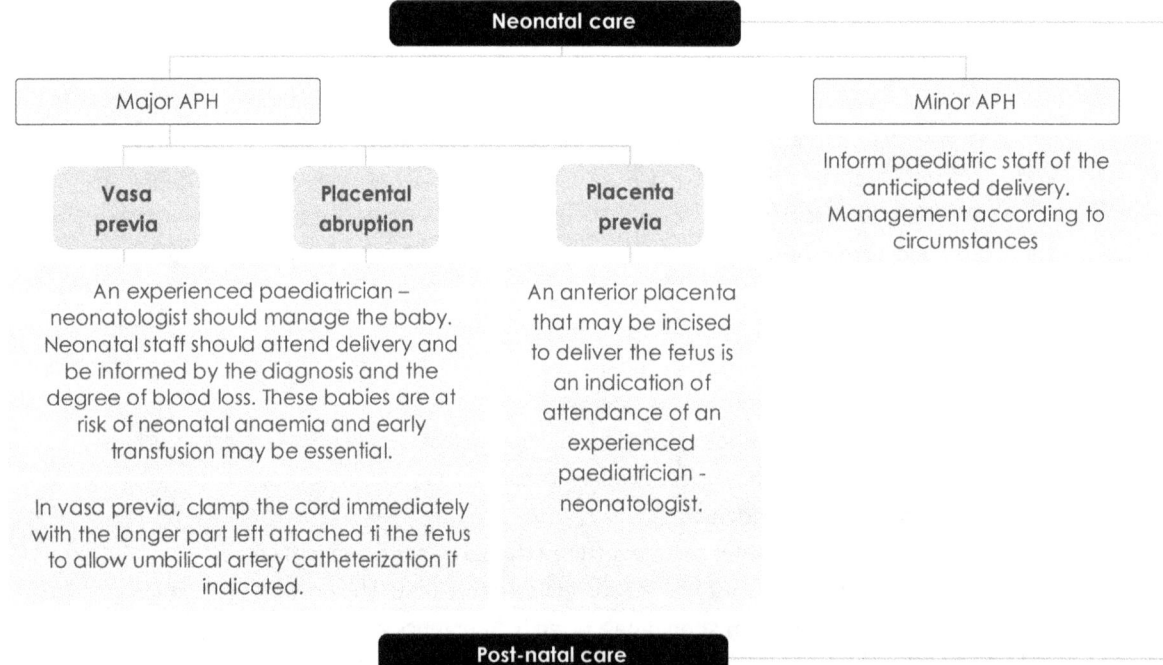

Major APH

| Vasa previa | Placental abruption | Placenta previa |

An experienced paediatrician – neonatologist should manage the baby. Neonatal staff should attend delivery and be informed by the diagnosis and the degree of blood loss. These babies are at risk of neonatal anaemia and early transfusion may be essential.

In vasa previa, clamp the cord immediately with the longer part left attached ti the fetus to allow umbilical artery catheterization if indicated.

An anterior placenta that may be incised to deliver the fetus is an indication of attendance of an experienced paediatrician - neonatologist.

Minor APH

Inform paediatric staff of the anticipated delivery. Management according to circumstances

Post-natal care

Contact numbers should be available during the postnatal care for medical and psychological support.
A follow-up visit 4 to 6 weeks postnatal should be offered.

Management of complications

Massive APH

The team

A consultant obstetrician, anaesthetist, haematologist and midwifery labour ward coordinator. Laboratory staff and portering staff is notified.

A Airway established.

B Breathing supported.

C Circulation supported.

Transfusion and circulation support are the same like in postpartum haemorrhage. Packed RBCs are associated with higher risk of acute tubular necrosis while whole blood transfusion is associated with higher risk of pulmonary edema.

Coagulopathy

DIC suspicion (should be considered with massive haemorrhage)

Platelet count and coagulation studies requested

Awaiting results

4 units of FFP (1 liter) and 10 units of cryoprecipitate (2 packs) empirically

Management according to the results

On anticoagulant therapy

Women on antenatal anti-coagulant therapy should stop therapy if they experience any vaginal bleeding. She should be referred immediately and assessed on hospital admission. Any further doses should be given after consultation of medical staff.
Women at high risk of haemorrhage and that are essentially in need for heparin therapy should use continuous IV unfractionated heparin infusion until the risk is resolved.

Fact Box: Counseling of women with antepartum haemorrhage

- **Antepartum counseling:** the mode of delivery, risk of haemorrhage, the possible need of blood transfusion and major surgical interventions including hysterectomy should be discussed with the woman and to be documented before delivery.
- **Consent for Cesarean section (particularly in placenta previa):**
  Prior to Cesarean section consent, any woman should understand:
  - The general risks of caesarean section and the specific risks in relation to placenta praevia particularly the risk of massive obstetric haemorrhage (12 times more).
  - The need for blood transfusion.
  - The chance of hysterectomy.

A consultant obstetrician should discuss the risks and treatment options with women with suspected placenta praevia accreta. Treatment plan is agreed and documents including:
  - The anticipated skin and uterine incisions.
  - Trial for conservative management of the placenta versus straight performance of hysterectomy if accreta is confirmed at surgery.
  - Additional interventions for massive haemorrhage should also be discussed including cell salvage and interventional radiology.

Prediction and prevention

Prediction

Placental abruption

70% of cases of placental abruption occur in low-risk women. So, APH cannot be clinically predicted.

Placenta previa

Clinical suspicion

- **Bleeding during pregnancy:** painless causeless bleeding (but may be provoked by sexual intercourse) after 20 weeks of pregnancy.
- **Fetal lie or presentation:** is abnormal. High presenting part is felt at term.

Ultrasound detection

Localization of placental site during routine anomaly scan (20 weeks)

Trans-abdominal ultrasound suggests placenta previa (PP)?

Trans-vaginal ultrasound
(To confirm the diagnosis specially if posterior)

Asymptomatic PP major?	**Asymptomatic PP minor?**
Repeat trans-vaginal Ultrasonography at 32 weeks	**Repeat trans-vaginal Ultrasonography at 36 weeks**

The diagnosis of placenta previa is persistent in only 11% of women (versus 50% in the presence on uterine scar). Color Doppler ultrasound is indicated in placenta previa anterior with previous uterine scar (risk of accreta).

Prevention

Placental abruption

- **Smoking cessation:** no evidence of prevention yet.
- **Cocaine and amphetamine cessation:** the evidence in prevention is lacking.
- **Folic acid supplements in pregnancy:** the evidence is controversial.
- **Antithrombotic therapy:** for women with thrombophilia. Initial results are promising.

Placenta previa

- **Vaginal and rectal examination:** should be avoided in women with placenta previa.
- **Penetrative sexual intercourse:** is better avoided.
- **Cervical cerclage:** there is no evidence to support its use in placenta previa.
- **Prophylactic tocolysis:** has no rule for prevention of bleeding in women with placenta previa.

Appendix I | **Placenta accreta**

Definition

Placenta accreta is a wide term that describes morbidly adherent placenta which include placenta accreta (penetrates through the decidua basalis), placenta increta (penetrates into the myometrium) and placenta percreta (penetrates through the myometrium to reach the peritoneum).

Diagnosis

A woman with previous uterine scar

Ultrasound screening (at 18-20^{+6} weeks)

Anterior placenta previa or a placenta situated over the scar

Ultrasound re-evaluation at 32 weeks

MRI in equivocal cases

Suggestive findings

Grayscale ultrasound	• Loss of the retroplacental sonolucent zone • Irregular retroplacental sonolucent zone • Thinning or disruption of the hyperechoic serosa–bladder interface • Presence of focal exophytic masses invading the urinary bladder • Abnormal placental lacunae.
Color Doppler ultrasound	• Diffuse or focal lacunar flow. • Vascular lakes with turbulent flow (peak systolic velocity over 15 cm/s). • Hypervascularity of serosa–bladder interface • Markedly dilated vessels over peripheral subplacental zone.
3D power Doppler ultrasound	• *Basal view:* numerous coherent vessels involving the whole uterine serosa–bladder junction. • *Lateral view:* Hypervascularity and inseparable cotyledonal and intervillous circulations, chaotic branching, detour vessels.
Magnetic resonance imaging (MRI)	• Uterine bulging • Heterogeneous signal intensity within the placenta • Dark intraplacental bands on T2-weighted imaging.

Intra-operative assessment

The presence of an abnormally adherent placenta at the time of Cesarean section is the only definitive diagnosis

Management

```
Suspected placenta accreta
```

Elective Cesarean section at 36-37 weeks

Delivery is planned. The most senior consultant is available. Other relative specialists should be notified.

Skin incision

A low transverse skin incision if the anterior upper margin of the placenta does not reach the upper segment of the uterus.

A midline skin incision if the anterior upper margin of placenta extending high towards the level of the umbilicus.

Incise the uterus away from the placenta site. Deliver the baby without disturbing the placenta.

Delivery of the placenta after the baby is out (definitive diagnosis of accreta)

If the placenta does not separate	**If the placenta partially separates**	**If the placenta completely separates**
Leave it in place and close the uterus or proceed to hysterectomy (aggressive trials to remove the placenta are associated with massive bleeding)	Remove the separated part. Adherent portion can be left in place and bleeding is dealt with according to the usual protocols (bleeding may be massive).	Remove the placenta as usual. Bleeding may continue from the placental bed and it needs to be managed according to the usual protocols.

Management of the possible massive haemorrhage

- **Calling for extra-help:** is the first step. There is no place for 'losing face' thinking.
- **Uterotonic agents:** should be considered.
- **Temporary bimanual compression:** or even aortic compression until help is available.
- **Specific approachs:** B-Lynch suture, uterine and internal iliac artery ligation.
    - Uterine and vaginal packing with gauze.
    - Balloon tamponade.
    - The B-Lynch suture/vertical compression sutures.
    - Suturing an inverted lip of cervix over the bleeding placenta bed.
    - Uterine and internal iliac artery ligation.
- **Interventional radiology:** facilities should be available specially if placenta accreta is suspected and the woman refuses blood transfusion.
  Prophylactic catheter placement for balloon occlusion or in readiness for embolisation needs further evaluation. There may be failure, post-removal bleeding or popliteal arterial thrombus.
- **Hysterectomy:** is the definitive last option

Follow up

- If a part or the whole placenta is left during Cesarean section, the woman is at risk of bleeding and infection. Prophylactic antibiotics immediately postpartum may reduce the risk:
  - The risk of bleeding is 35%.
  - The risk of infection is 18%.
  - The risk of DIC is 7%.
- Methotrexate and arterial embolisation do not reduce the risk. Both are not recommended as a routine.
- Follow-up of the woman using:
  - *Serum beta-hCG:* weekly measurement is to check that it is falling. However, low levels do not guarantee complete placental resolution.
  - *Ultrasound assessment:* to confirm complete resolution based on hCG measurements.

There is no adequate data about future pregnancy and the possible risk of recurrence of placenta accreta.

| Appendix II | Vasa previa |

Definition

Vasa praevia is a condition in which fetal vessels pass through the membranes over the region of the internal cervical os below the fetal presenting part. So it is unprotected by either the placental tissue or the umbilical cord.
This condition is met only once in 2000 to 6000 pregnancies.

Risk factors

- Placental anomalies such as a bilobed placenta or succenturiate lobes.
- A low-lying placenta in the second trimester.
- Multiple pregnancy.
- In vitro fertilization: the incidence of vasa praevia is 1 in 300. The association is not yet clearly explained.

Types

| Vasa previa type 1 | Vasa previa secondary to a velamentous cord insertion in a single or bilobed placenta. |
| Vasa previa type 2 | Vasa previa from fetal vessels passing between lobes of a placenta with one or more accessory lobes. |

Complications

- Vasa praevia threatens the fetus rather than the mother that almost has no risk.
- Vasa previa carries the risk of fetal mortality. The mortality rate is 60% versus 97% if it diagnosed antenatally.

Diagnosis

Antenatal diagnosis

- **Clinical diagnosis:** there is no clinical method to diagnose vasa previa antenatally if there is no vaginal bleeding (Bleeding rarely occurs with intact membranes).
- **Ultrasonographic diagnosis:** suspicious cases (e.g. placental abnormalities) can be confirmed by transvaginal color Doppler scan (not done routinely).
- **Cardiotocographic diagnosis:** pathological changes or even sinusoidal pattern may be associated with vasa previa (not specific).

Intrapartum diagnosis

- **Before membrane rupture:** clinical diagnosis may occasionally be achieved bt palpating the apparent vessels through the membranes. This can be confirmed by direct visualization using an amnioscope.
- **After membrane rupture:** sudden vaginal bleeding following membrane rupture with fetal compromise (decelerations, bradycardia, sinusoidal trace or demise). No trial to confirm diagnosis is made and immediate management is indicated.

Postpartum diagnosis

Simple examination confirms the presence of apparent vessels but cannot confirm its relation to the internal os.

Differentiation

Tests to differentiate between vasa previa and other causes of APH is based on the fact that vasa previa is the only cause of APH that is totally fetal in origin. So differentiation between fetal and maternal blood helps to confirm or exclude vasa previa. Unfortunately, these tests are not practical because there is no time to be performed after bleeding starts.

The Kleihauer–Bekte test and haemoglobin electrophoresis

- Both can identify fetal cells in vaginal blood loss. They detect fetal haemoglobin concentrations as low as 0.01%.
- The disadvantage of both is that they are time consuming.

A simple bedside test

0.14 M sodium hydroxide solution is added to the sample. It normally denatures adult haemoglobin (becomes brownish green) rather than fetal haemoglobin (remains red).

This method may be more applicable but it requires further evaluation.

Management

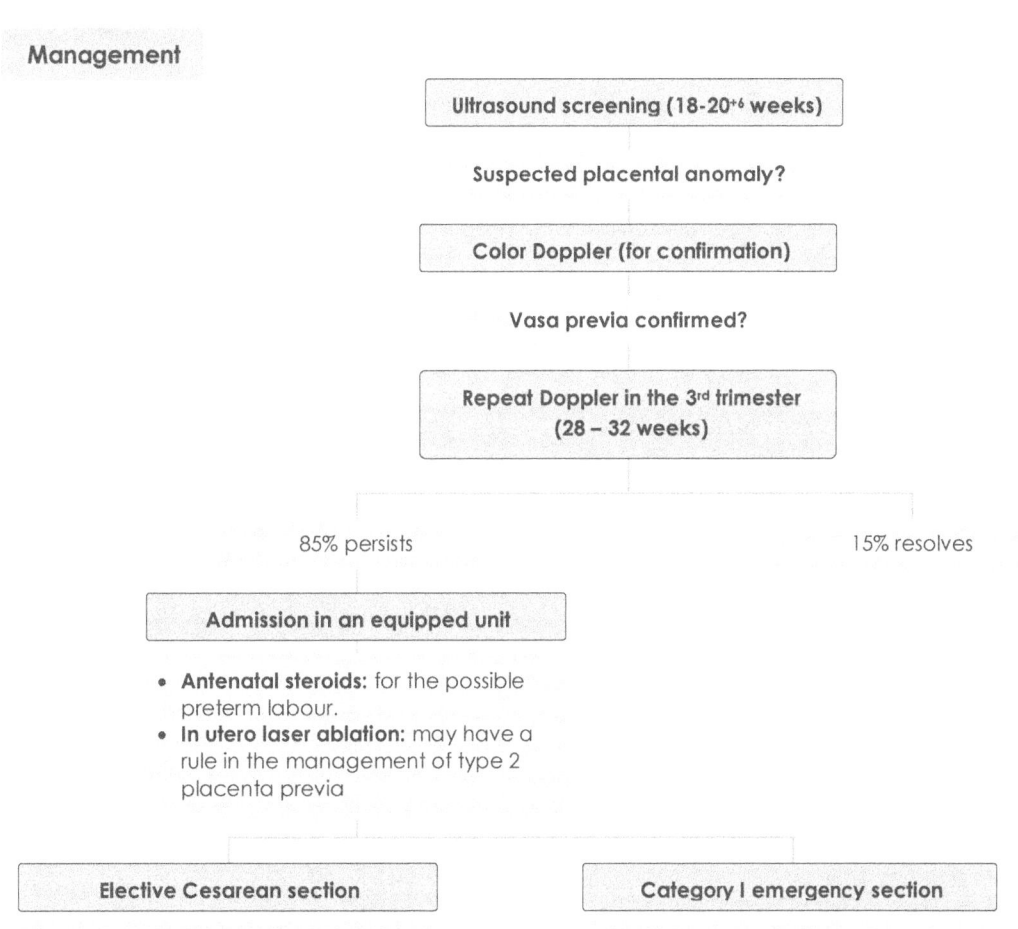

Ultrasound screening (18-20^{+6} weeks)

Suspected placental anomaly?

Color Doppler (for confirmation)

Vasa previa confirmed?

Repeat Doppler in the 3rd trimester (28 – 32 weeks)

85% persists   15% resolves

Admission in an equipped unit

- **Antenatal steroids:** for the possible preterm labour.
- **In utero laser ablation:** may have a rule in the management of type 2 placenta previa

Elective Cesarean section	Category I emergency section
It is carried out between 35 and 37 weeks of gestation	It is carried out if bleeding starts at any time

CHAPTER 5
MEDICAL DISORDERS

STATION 5: MEDICAL DISORDERS WITH PREGNANCY

Hypertensive disorders with pregnancy

BACKGROUND   *What obstetrician should know about hypertension with pregnancy*

Definitions

Hypertension with pregnancy is defined as a diastolic blood pressure ≥ 90 mmHg or systolic blood pressure ≥ 140 mmHg (on two occasions more than 4 hours apart) or a single diastolic blood pressure ≥ 110 mmHg.

Degrees

Mild hypertension

Diastolic blood pressure 90–99 mmHg or systolic blood pressure 140–149 mmHg

Moderate hypertension

Diastolic blood pressure 100–109 mmHg or systolic blood pressure 150–159 mmHg

Severe hypertension

Diastolic blood pressure ≥ 110 mmHg or systolic blood pressure ≥ 160 mmHg

Classification

Chronic hypertension

It refers to hypertension present at booking visit, before 20 weeks or if the woman is already diagnosed and on treatment when referred for antenatal care.

Gestational hypertension

New hypertension diagnosed after 20 weeks of gestation without significant proteinuria

Pre-eclampsia

New hypertension diagnosed after 20 weeks of gestation with significant proteinuria

Mild preeclampsia

Pre-eclampsia with mild hypertension diagnosed after 20 weeks of gestation with significant proteinuria

Severe preeclampsia

Pre-eclampsia with severe hypertension and/or symptoms, biochemical or haematological impairment.

Features of severe pre-eclampsia

Severe hypertension and proteinuria or mild/moderate hypertension and proteinuria with one of: severe headache, visual problems (blurring or flashing), severe pain below ribs or vomiting, papilloedema, clonus (≥ 3 beats), liver tenderness, HELLP syndrome, platelet count falls to < 100 x 109/litre or abnormal liver enzymes (ALT or AST rises to > 70 iu/litre).

Eclampsia

Preeclampsia complicated by convulsive condition

Incidence

- Hypertension affects 10% of pregnant women.
- Pre-eclampsia affects 4.1% of women in their first pregnancy and 1.7% in the second pregnancy.

Complications

Maternal

Short-term hazards

- **Maternal mortality:** it is the second commonest cause in UK. Intra-cranial haemorrhage is the commonest cause of death in preeclampsia.
- **Maternal morbidity:** it is responsible of 33% of severe maternal morbidity in the UK.

Cerebral hemorrhage
Placental abruption
HELLP syndrome
Acute renal failure
Eclampsia
Pulmonary edema

Long-term hazards

	Gestational hypertension	Pre-eclampsia	Severe pre-eclampsia
Recurrent Gestational hypertension	Risk of recurrence is 16-47%	Risk of recurrence is 13-53%	
Future Pre-eclampsia	Risk is 2-7%	Risk is 16% (no risk if pregnancy interval < 10 years)	55% (if woman delivers < 28 weeks), 25% (if she delivers < 34 weeks)
CV diseases	Increase risk of hypertension and its complications		
End stage kidney disease	Risk of recurrence is 16-47%	If no hypertension or proteinuria 6-8 weeks postnatal, relative risk increases but absolute risk is low (do not follow up)	

Fetal

- **Stillbirth:** preeclampsia is responsible for 5% of stillbirths in non-anomalous fetuses in the UK.
- **Pre-maturity:** it is responsible for 8-10% of preterm labour (10% of women with severe pre-eclampsia deliver before 34 weeks and 50% give birth before 37 weeks).
- **Fetal growth restriction:** FGR affects 25% of preterm births and 15-20% of term births in women with pre-eclampsia.

APPROACH   *How obstetricians should deal with hypertension with pregnancy*

First   Women at risk of hypertension with pregnancy (risk reduction)

Assessment at booking

Fetal risk

- Previous severe eclampsia
- Previous pre-eclampsia that indicates preterm delivery < 34 weeks
- Previous pre-eclampsia with neonatal birth weight < 10th centile.
- Previous intrauterine death
- Previous placental abruption

Maternal risk

Low risk

No high or moderate risk factor is identified by history, general and obstetric assessment

Moderate risk

- First pregnancy
- Age ≥ 40 years
- Pregnancy interval > 10 years
- BMI ≥ 35 kg/m2 at first visit
- Family history of pre-eclampsia
- Multiple pregnancy

High risk

- Previous hypertensive disease in pregnancy
- Chronic kidney disease
- Autoimmune disease e.g. SLE or antiphospholipid syndrome
- Type 1 or 2 diabetes
- Chronic hypertension

Fetal growth and amniotic fluid volume assessment using ultrasound plus Umbilical artery Doppler velocimetry
It starts at 28–30 weeks (or at least 2 weeks before previous gestational age of the onset of hypertensive disorder if earlier than 28 weeks)

Repeat 4 weeks later

Measurement of blood pressure and assessment of proteinuria during each antenatal care visit

Life style modification during pregnancy (rest, exercise and work)*

Ask women to contact health care professional immediately if they experience any symptoms of severe preeclampsia **

2 moderate risk factors (at least)

1 high risk factor (at least)

The same percussions as low risk women

Plus

Counsel women to use aspirin (75 mg/day) from 12 weeks until birth – Informed consent is required because this indication is unlicensed.

Plus

Cardiotocography when fetal activity is reduced

Do not recommend the following to protect against hypertension during pregnancy
- Drugs including nitric oxide donors, diuretics, progesterone and LMW heparin.
- Supplements e.g. magnesium, folic acid, antioxidants (vitamins C and E), fish or algal oils, or garlic.
- Diet modification e.g. restricting salt intake.

* See under section: antenatal care
** Severe headache, epigastric pain, visual problems (flushing, blurring), vomiting, sudden face or limb swelling

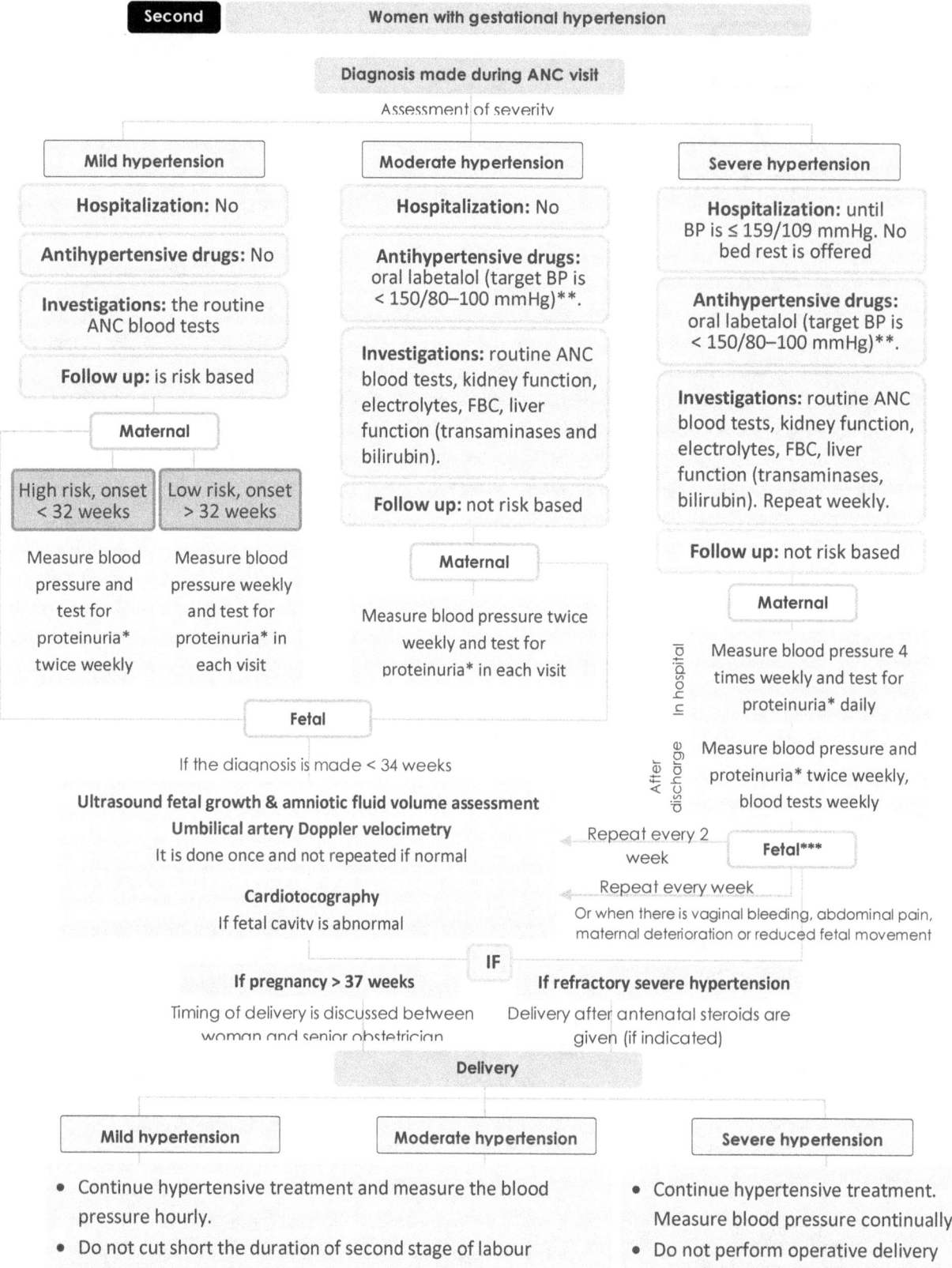

Second   Women with gestational hypertension

Diagnosis made during ANC visit

Assessment of severity

Mild hypertension

Hospitalization: No

Antihypertensive drugs: No

Investigations: the routine ANC blood tests

Follow up: is risk based

Maternal

High risk, onset < 32 weeks	Low risk, onset > 32 weeks
Measure blood pressure and test for proteinuria* twice weekly	Measure blood pressure weekly and test for proteinuria* in each visit

Moderate hypertension

Hospitalization: No

Antihypertensive drugs: oral labetalol (target BP is < 150/80–100 mmHg)**.

Investigations: routine ANC blood tests, kidney function, electrolytes, FBC, liver function (transaminases and bilirubin).

Follow up: not risk based

Maternal

Measure blood pressure twice weekly and test for proteinuria* in each visit

Severe hypertension

Hospitalization: until BP is ≤ 159/109 mmHg. No bed rest is offered

Antihypertensive drugs: oral labetalol (target BP is < 150/80–100 mmHg)**.

Investigations: routine ANC blood tests, kidney function, electrolytes, FBC, liver function (transaminases, bilirubin). Repeat weekly.

Follow up: not risk based

Maternal

In hospital — Measure blood pressure 4 times weekly and test for proteinuria* daily

After discharge — Measure blood pressure and proteinuria* twice weekly, blood tests weekly

Fetal

If the diagnosis is made < 34 weeks

Ultrasound fetal growth & amniotic fluid volume assessment
Umbilical artery Doppler velocimetry
It is done once and not repeated if normal

Cardiotocography
If fetal cavity is abnormal

Repeat every 2 week

Repeat every week

Fetal*

Or when there is vaginal bleeding, abdominal pain, maternal deterioration or reduced fetal movement

IF

If pregnancy > 37 weeks

Timing of delivery is discussed between woman and senior obstetrician

If refractory severe hypertension

Delivery after antenatal steroids are given (if indicated)

Delivery

Mild hypertension   **Moderate hypertension**   **Severe hypertension**

- Continue hypertensive treatment and measure the blood pressure hourly.
- Do not cut short the duration of second stage of labour routinely if BP stable.

- Continue hypertensive treatment. Measure blood pressure continually
- Do not perform operative delivery unless BP is not controlled by drugs

* Test for proteinuria using an automated reagent-strip reading device or urinary protein:creatinine ratio.
** Methyldopa and Nifedipine are another alternatives.
*** A written care plan of fetal monitoring, steroids and time for neonologist/anesthetist discussion is provided

Postnatal care

Maternal care

Modification of hypertensive drugs

If woman is not on treatment	If woman is on treatment
Hypertensive treatment only if ≥ 150/100 mmHg.	Continue. Methyldopa is stopped within 2 days

Follow up blood pressure

BP is measured daily for 2 days
Then
Once 3-5 days postpartum

If < 130/80	If < 140/90
Reduce hypertensive treatment	Consider treatment reduction

Referral to community care

- Who will follow-up the woman
- Frequency of assessment of blood pressure and when to reduce or stop treatment
- Indications for referral to primary care for blood pressure review.

Treatment continues ? → Offer medical review 2 weeks postnatal

Offer medical review 6-8 weeks postnatal

Referral to hypertension specialist ← Treatment continues ?

Neonatal care

Assessment of neonatal well being and adequacy of breast-feeding daily for 2 days

Avoid the use of diuretics during breast feeding

Third   Women with chronic hypertension

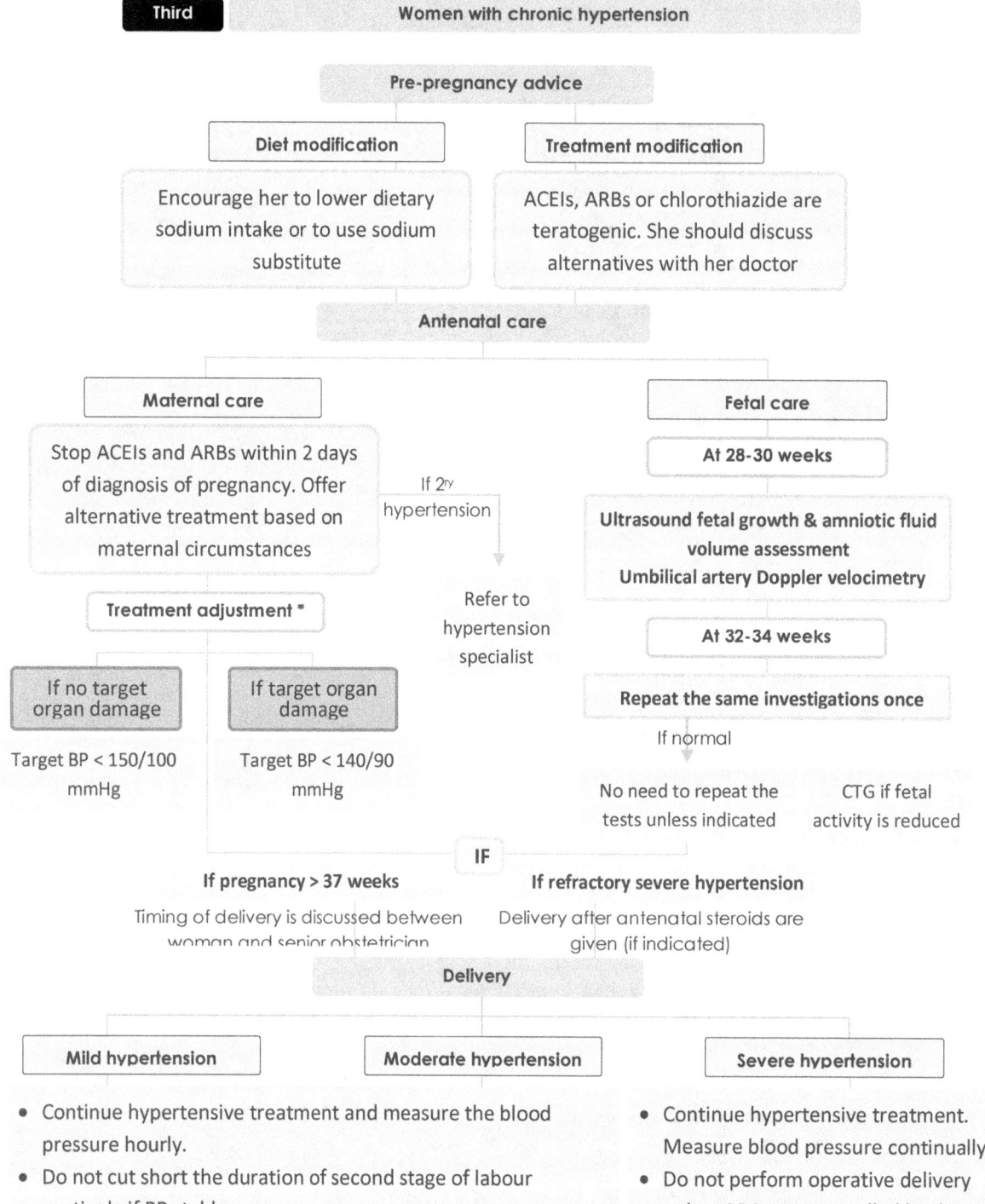

Pre-pregnancy advice

Diet modification

Encourage her to lower dietary sodium intake or to use sodium substitute

Treatment modification

ACEIs, ARBs or chlorothiazide are teratogenic. She should discuss alternatives with her doctor

Antenatal care

Maternal care

Stop ACEIs and ARBs within 2 days of diagnosis of pregnancy. Offer alternative treatment based on maternal circumstances

If 2ry hypertension

Refer to hypertension specialist

Treatment adjustment *

If no target organ damage

If target organ damage

Target BP < 150/100 mmHg

Target BP < 140/90 mmHg

Fetal care

At 28-30 weeks

Ultrasound fetal growth & amniotic fluid volume assessment
Umbilical artery Doppler velocimetry

At 32-34 weeks

Repeat the same investigations once

If normal

No need to repeat the tests unless indicated

CTG if fetal activity is reduced

IF

If pregnancy > 37 weeks

Timing of delivery is discussed between woman and senior obstetrician

If refractory severe hypertension

Delivery after antenatal steroids are given (if indicated)

Delivery

Mild hypertension

- Continue hypertensive treatment and measure the blood pressure hourly.
- Do not cut short the duration of second stage of labour routinely if BP stable.

Moderate hypertension

Severe hypertension

- Continue hypertensive treatment. Measure blood pressure continually
- Do not perform operative delivery unless BP is not controlled by drugs

* Do not lower the diastolic blood pressure below 80 mmHg

Postnatal care

Maternal care

Modification of hypertensive drugs

If woman is on Methyldopa	If woman is on other drugs
Stop within 2 days. Restart pre-pregnancy treatment	Continue antenatal hypertensive treatment

Follow up blood pressure

BP is measured daily for 2 days
Then
Once 3-5 days postpartum

Ensure blood pressure < 140/90

Adjust long term treatment 2 weeks postnatal

Offer medical review 6-8 weeks postnatal by the pre-pregnancy

Neonatal care

Assessment of neonatal well being and adequacy of breast-feeding daily for 2 days

Avoid the use of diuretics during breast feeding

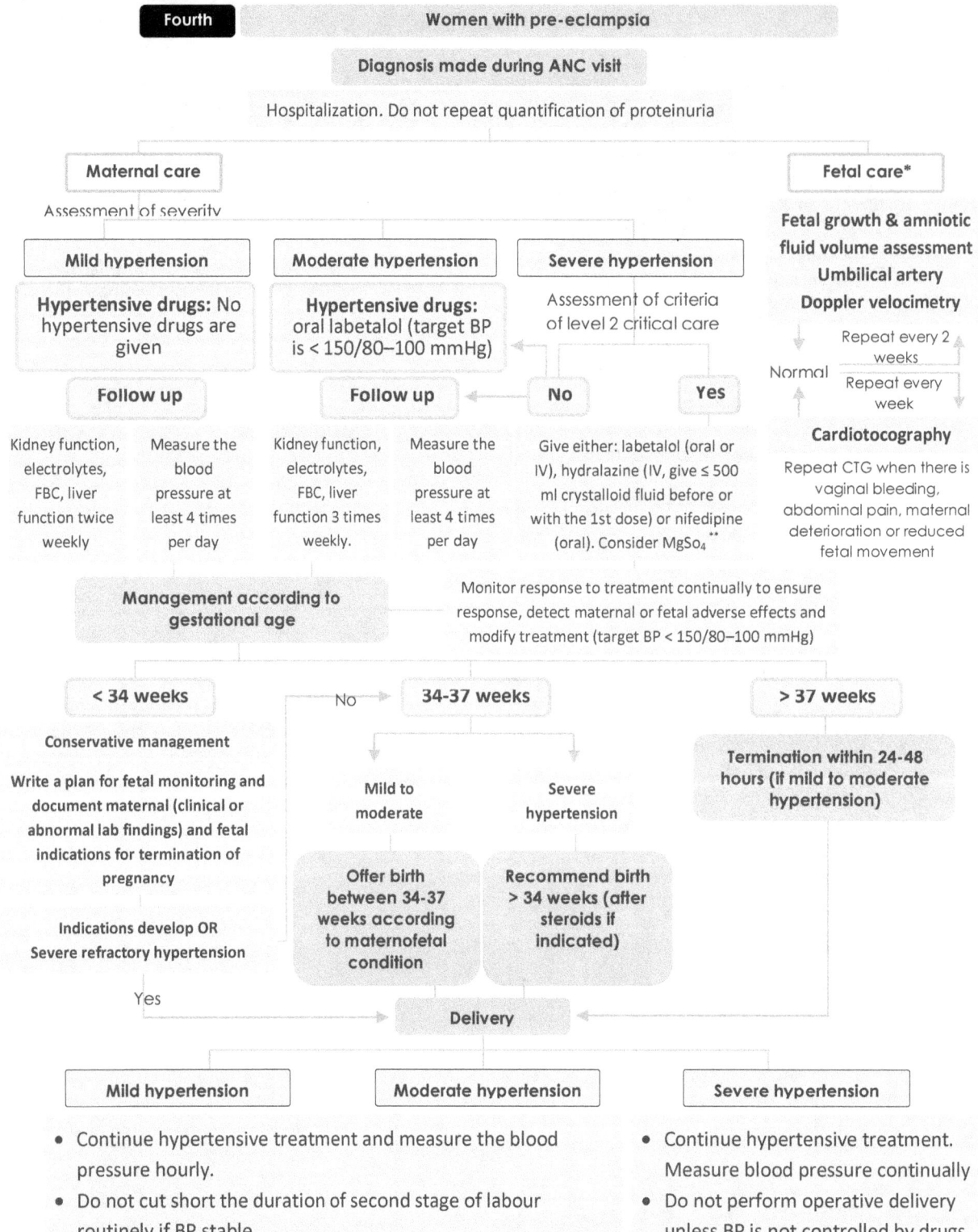

Fourth — Women with pre-eclampsia

Diagnosis made during ANC visit

Hospitalization. Do not repeat quantification of proteinuria

Maternal care — **Fetal care***

Assessment of severity

Mild hypertension | **Moderate hypertension** | **Severe hypertension**

Hypertensive drugs: No hypertensive drugs are given

Hypertensive drugs: oral labetalol (target BP is < 150/80–100 mmHg)

Assessment of criteria of level 2 critical care

No / **Yes**

Follow up | **Follow up**

Kidney function, electrolytes, FBC, liver function twice weekly | Measure the blood pressure at least 4 times per day | Kidney function, electrolytes, FBC, liver function 3 times weekly. | Measure the blood pressure at least 4 times per day | Give either: labetalol (oral or IV), hydralazine (IV, give ≤ 500 ml crystalloid fluid before or with the 1st dose) or nifedipine (oral). Consider MgSo$_4$**

Fetal growth & amniotic fluid volume assessment
Umbilical artery Doppler velocimetry

Normal — Repeat every 2 weeks / Repeat every week

Cardiotocography

Repeat CTG when there is vaginal bleeding, abdominal pain, maternal deterioration or reduced fetal movement

Management according to gestational age

Monitor response to treatment continually to ensure response, detect maternal or fetal adverse effects and modify treatment (target BP < 150/80–100 mmHg)

< 34 weeks   No → **34-37 weeks**   **> 37 weeks**

Conservative management

Write a plan for fetal monitoring and document maternal (clinical or abnormal lab findings) and fetal indications for termination of pregnancy

Indications develop OR Severe refractory hypertension

Yes

Mild to moderate | Severe hypertension

Offer birth between 34-37 weeks according to maternofetal condition | **Recommend birth > 34 weeks (after steroids if indicated)**

Termination within 24-48 hours (if mild to moderate hypertension)

Delivery

Mild hypertension | **Moderate hypertension** | **Severe hypertension**

- Continue hypertensive treatment and measure the blood pressure hourly.
- Do not cut short the duration of second stage of labour routinely if BP stable.

- Continue hypertensive treatment. Measure blood pressure continually
- Do not perform operative delivery unless BP is not controlled by drugs

---

* A written care plan of fetal monitoring, steroids and time for neonologist/anesthetist discussion is provided
** Magnesium sulfate:
- *Indications:*
  - If woman with severe hypertension or severe pre-eclampsia has or previously had eclamptic fit.
  - If birth planned within 24 hours in woman with severe pre-eclampsia.
- *Regimen:* Loading dose of 4 g given intravenously over 5 minutes, followed by infusion of 1 g/hour for 24 hours. Further dose of 2–4 g given over 5 minutes if recurrent seizures.

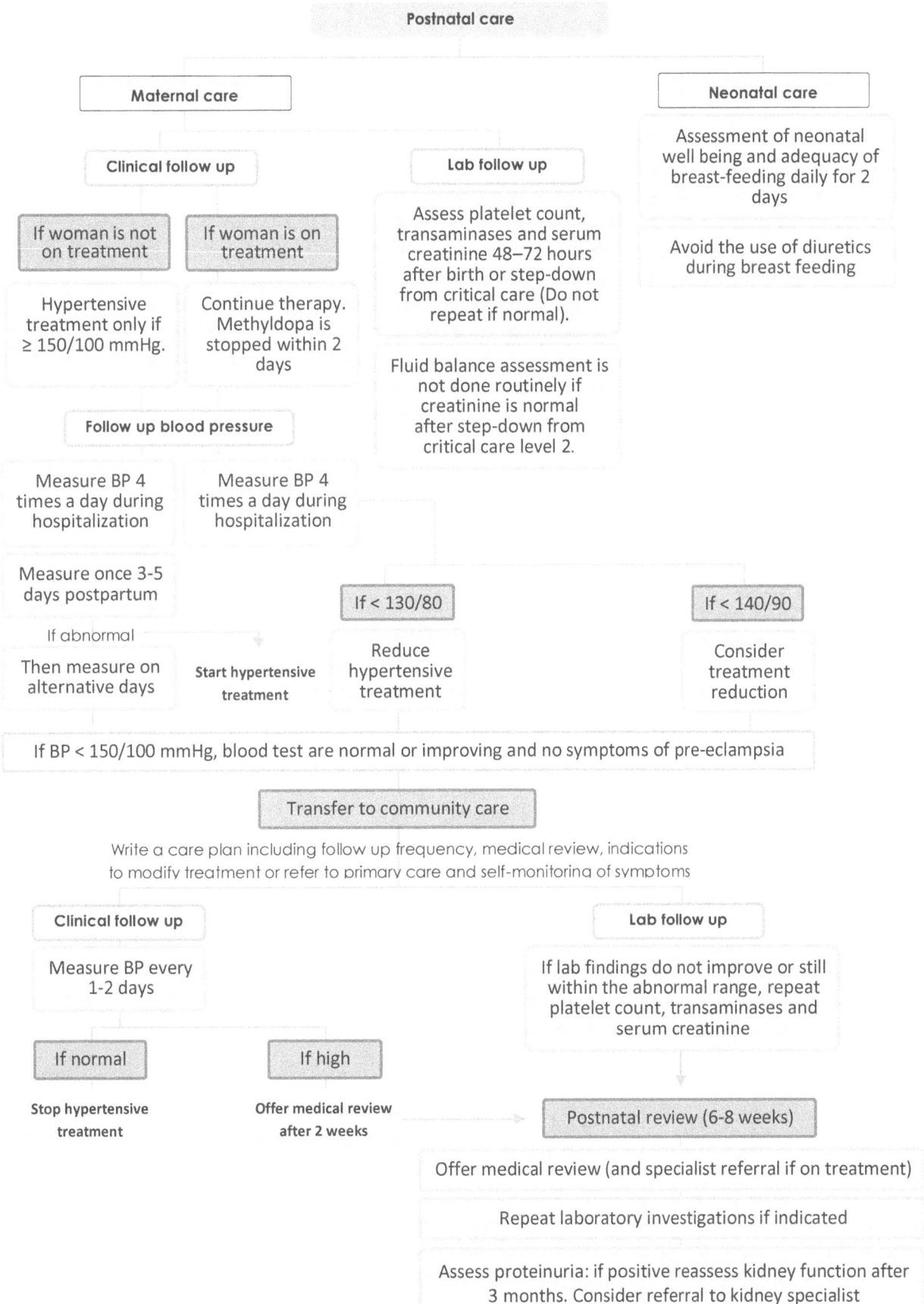

Postnatal care

Maternal care

Neonatal care

Assessment of neonatal well being and adequacy of breast-feeding daily for 2 days

Avoid the use of diuretics during breast feeding

Clinical follow up

Lab follow up

If woman is not on treatment

If woman is on treatment

Assess platelet count, transaminases and serum creatinine 48–72 hours after birth or step-down from critical care (Do not repeat if normal).

Hypertensive treatment only if ≥ 150/100 mmHg.

Continue therapy. Methyldopa is stopped within 2 days

Fluid balance assessment is not done routinely if creatinine is normal after step-down from critical care level 2.

Follow up blood pressure

Measure BP 4 times a day during hospitalization

Measure BP 4 times a day during hospitalization

Measure once 3-5 days postpartum

If < 130/80

If < 140/90

If abnormal

Then measure on alternative days

Start hypertensive treatment

Reduce hypertensive treatment

Consider treatment reduction

If BP < 150/100 mmHg, blood test are normal or improving and no symptoms of pre-eclampsia

Transfer to community care

Write a care plan including follow up frequency, medical review, indications to modify treatment or refer to primary care and self-monitoring of symptoms

Clinical follow up

Lab follow up

Measure BP every 1-2 days

If lab findings do not improve or still within the abnormal range, repeat platelet count, transaminases and serum creatinine

If normal

If high

Stop hypertensive treatment

Offer medical review after 2 weeks

Postnatal review (6-8 weeks)

Offer medical review (and specialist referral if on treatment)

Repeat laboratory investigations if indicated

Assess proteinuria: if positive reassess kidney function after 3 months. Consider referral to kidney specialist

Criteria for referral to critical care in women with severe pre-eclampsia	
Level 1 care	• Pre-eclampsia with mild or moderate hypertension. • Conservative antenatal management of severe preterm hypertension. • Step-down treatment after the birth.

Level 2 care	• Step-down from level 3 or severe
	• pre-eclampsia with one of the following:
	  ▪ Eclampsia
	  ▪ HELLP syndrome
	  ▪ Haemorrhage
	  ▪ Hyperkalaemia
	  ▪ Severe oliguria
	  ▪ Coagulation support
	  ▪ Intravenous antihypertensive treatment
	  ▪ Initial stabilisation of severe hypertension
	  ▪ Cardiac failure
	  ▪ Abnormal neurology.

Level 3 care	Severe pre-eclampsia that necessitates ventilation.

Appendix I   **Clinical assessment: blood pressure and proteinuria**

Blood pressure assessment

The woman is prepared in the sitting or semi-reclining position. The arm is set at the level of the heart.

Remove tight clothes and let the arm be relaxed and supported.

Use an appropriate size cuff. This depends on the circumference of the arm.

Upper arm circumference 18-22cm: Small cuff

Upper arm circumference 23 – 32 cm: Standard (13x23cm) adult cuff

Upper arm circumference 33 – 41 cm: Large (33x15 cm) adult cuff

Upper arm circumference > 41 cm: Thigh (18x36cm)

Obtain an estimated systolic pressure by palpation, to avoid auscultatory gap.

Inflate the cuff to 20–30 mmHg above palpated systolic blood pressure.

Lower the column slowly by 2 mmHg/second or beat and read the blood pressure to the nearest 2 mmHg

Measure the diastolic pressure at Korotkoff phase V. However, in 15% of pregnant women, the diastolic pressure falls to 0 before the sound disappears, then both phase IV and phase V readings should be recorded (e.g. 132/88/0 mmHg).

Assessment of proteinuria

Use an automated reagent-strip reading device (or a spot urinary protein:creatinine ratio) in secondary care.

If the automated reagent-strip reading device is positive for proteinuria (≥ 1+), use either a spot urinary protein:creatinine ratio or 24-hour urine collection to quantify proteinuria.

Urinary protein:creatinine ratio > 30 mg/mmol = significant proteinuria

A validated 24-hour urine collection with > 300 mg protein = significant proteinuria

| Appendix II | **Drug index of obstetric hypertension** |

Fluid balance and volume expansion

The following is to be considered in women with severe pre-eclampsia:
- Do not preload with intravenous fluids before low-dose epidural analgesia and combined spinal/epidural analgesia are established.
- A maintenance fluid is limited to 80 ml/hour unless there are other losses (e.g. haemorrhage).
- Volume expansion is indicated if hydralazine is given for severe hypertension.

Antenatal steroids

- **Indications:**
  - If birth is expected within 7 days.
  - There is no rule for steroids in the treatment of HELLP syndrome.
- **Regimens:**
  - 2 doses of betamethasone (12 mg intramuscularly) 24 hours apart between 24 and 34 weeks
  - Consider giving 2 doses betamethasone (12 mg intramuscularly) 24 hours apart at 35–36 weeks.
  - Informed consent is obtained and documented (unlicensed indication).

ACE inhibitors

- **Captopril:**
  - It is already used in UK postnatal obstetric practice.
  - It is contraindicated in the second and third trimesters of pregnancy and in lactation. It is not recommended during the first trimester of pregnancy.
  - Informed consent is obtained and documented in these situations.
- **Enalapril:**
  - It is already used widely in UK postnatal obstetric practice.
  - It is contraindicated in the second and third trimesters of pregnancy. It is not recommended during the first trimester of pregnancy or in breast-feeding for preterm infants and for the first few weeks after delivery.
  - Informed consent is obtained and documented in these situations.

Sympatholytics

- **Labetalol:**
  - It is licensed for the treatment of hypertension even during pregnancy.
  - It should only be used during the first trimester of pregnancy if the potential benefit outweighs the potential risk. Breastfeeding is not recommended.
  - Informed consent is obtained and documented in these situations.
- **Methyldopa:**
  - It is licensed for the treatment of hypertension and is used widely in UK.
  - It is used in women who are, or may become, pregnant or who are breastfeeding only if the anticipated benefits be weighed against the risks.
  - Informed consent is obtained and documented in these situations.
- **Metoprolol/Atenolol:**
  - Both are licensed for the treatment of hypertension and are used widely in UK.
  - Metoprolol is used in women who are pregnant or breastfeeding if the anticipated benefit is weighed against the possible risks.
  - Atenolol is used in women who may become pregnant, in the first and second trimester of pregnancy or breastfeeding if the anticipated benefit is weighed against the possible risks.
  - Informed consent is obtained and documented in these situations.

Ca channel blockers	• **Nifedipine:** ▪ It is licensed for the treatment of hypertension and is already used widely in UK. ▪ It is contraindicated in pregnancy before week 20. It should not be used during the entire pregnancy or in women who may become pregnant. ▪ It should not be used during breastfeeding. ▪ Informed consent is obtained and documented in these situations.

STATION 5: MEDICAL DISORDERS WITH PREGNANCY

Diabetes in pregnancy

BACKGROUND   *What obstetrician should know about diabetes with pregnancy*

Classification

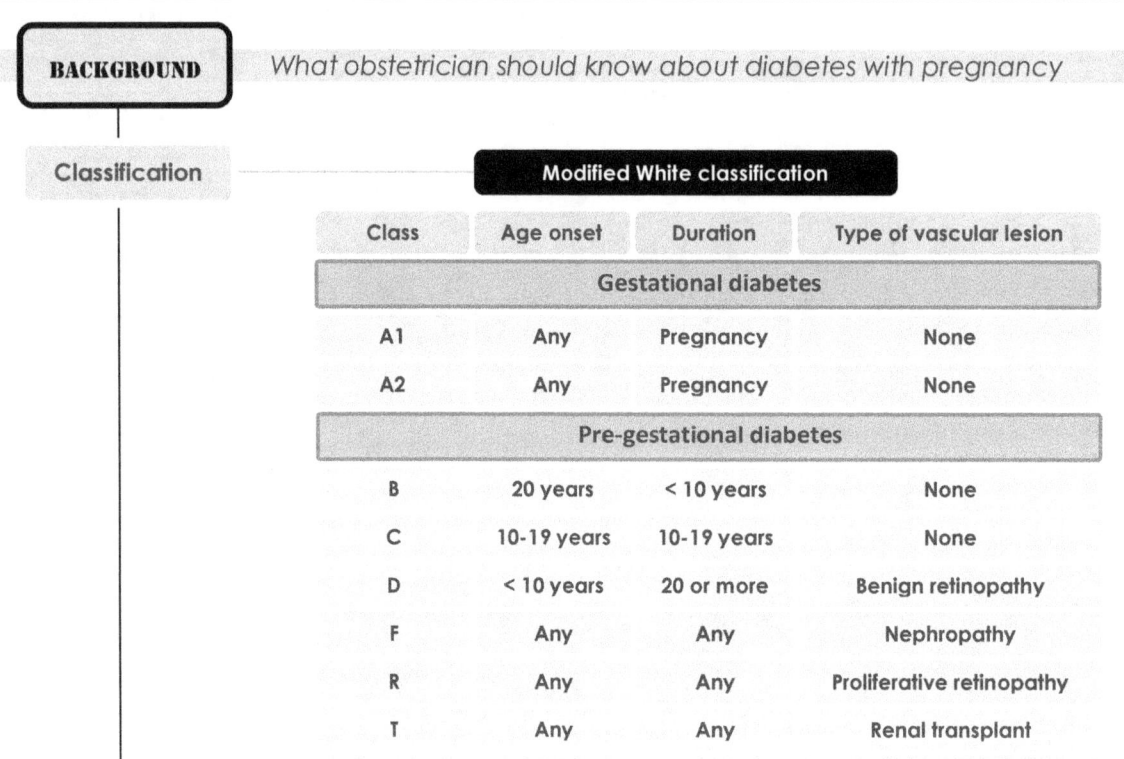

Class	Age onset	Duration	Type of vascular lesion
Gestational diabetes			
A1	Any	Pregnancy	None
A2	Any	Pregnancy	None
Pre-gestational diabetes			
B	20 years	< 10 years	None
C	10-19 years	10-19 years	None
D	< 10 years	20 or more	Benign retinopathy
F	Any	Any	Nephropathy
R	Any	Any	Proliferative retinopathy
T	Any	Any	Renal transplant
H	Any	Any	Coronary artery disease

Diabetes complicates 4/1000 pregnancies in the UK, pre-existing insulin-dependent diabetes mellitus represent the majority of cases.

Complications

- Fetal macrosomia
- Birth trauma (maternal and newborn)
- Induction of labour or caesarean section
- Miscarriage
- Congenital malformation
- Stillbirth
- Transient neonatal morbidity
- Neonatal death
- Obesity and/or diabetes in later life.

| APPROACH | *How obstetricians should deal with diabetes with pregnancy* |

Pre-gestational Diabetes

Pre-conception care

Inform on

The benefits of pre-conception glycaemic control and avoidance of unplanned pregnancy

The risks of diabetes in pregnancy and how to reduce them by proper glycaemic control

Diet and exercise. Reduction of body weight if her BMI is above 27 kg/m^2

The proper time to stop contraception

Pregnancy-related nausea and vomiting and the associated glycaemic control

Awareness of hypoglycaemia   Retinal and renal assessment

Offer

Diabetes structured education programme

Blood glucose meter for self-monitoring of glycaemic control

Ketone testing strips. Women with type 1 DM should use it if hyperglycaemic or feeing unwell

HbA1c monthly

Retinal assessment with mydriasis using tropicamide (if it is not carried out in previous 6 months)

Renal assessment (including microalbuminuria) before stopping contraception

IF

| Serum creatinine is 120 micromol/litre or more | The estimated glomerular filtration rate (eGFR) is < 45 ml/minute/1.73 m^2 |

Consider referral to a specialist (a nephrologist)

Review

The current treatment of diabetes according to the safety profile before and during pregnancy

Current treatment	Modified treatment
Oral hypoglycemics	Stop all except metformin/start insulin
Metformin	Continue instead of or with insulin
ACEIs, AT-II blockers, statins	Stop
Insulin	Rapid-acting insulin (aspart and lispro) is not evident to have obstetric adverse effects. Evidence about long acting insulin is limited. Isophane (NPH) insulin is the first-choice long-acting insulin during pregnancy.

The blood glucose target and monitoring of glucose level

Monthly HBA1C Reduction of HBA1C reduces the risk. If it is < 6.1 (if safe) is the target. HBA1C > 10 should not get pregnant	**Determine blood glucose target on individualized base** If a woman needs intense therapy, she needs to increase the frequency of monitoring (including fasting, pre- and postprandial levels). Rapid optimization is postponed until retinal assessment/treatment are done

Give

Folic acid 5 mg and continue after getting pregnant to the end of the first tremester

Stop contraception and plan for pregnancy

Pre-gestational Diabetes

Antenatal care

First appointment

Taking medical history

Retinal and renal assessment

They are indicated in the first appointment if they are not assessed in the last 12 months

Retinal assessment	**Renal assessment**
Retinal assessment is carried out by digital imaging with mydriasis using tropicamide to confirm/exclude diabetic retinopathy	• If serum creatinine ≥ 120 μmol/L or total protein excretion > 2 g/day: refer to specialist. • If proteinuria > 5gm/day: give thromboprophylaxis • Do not offer eGFR

Review medications (mentioned)

Diabetic monitoring

Glucose monitoring	**Ketone monitoring**
Determine individualised glucose targets for self-monitoring	Women with type 1 DM should be offered ketone testing strips if hyperglycemic or unwell

Glucose monitoring:

Monitor by fasting and 1-hour postprandial blood glucose levels after every meal	Assessment of HBA1c (it is not done routinely in the second or the third trimester)
Keep fasting blood glucose 3.5-5.9 mmol/litre & 1-hour postprandial glucose < 7.8 mmol/litre	If HBA1c is high, offer rapid optimization of blood glucose even in the presence of retinopathy

Ketone monitoring:

If suspected

Admit women immediately for level 2 critical care

Emergency advices (for insulin)

Women should be advised on the risk of hypoglycemia (specially in the first trimester). They should test their blood glucose before going to bed. Concentrated oral glucose and glucagon should be available. The family members should be aware of using them.

If multiple insulin injections are inadequate with significant hypoglycaemia

Consider insulin pump therapy

7-9 weeks	Trans-vaginal ultrasound is performed to confirm fetal viability and gestational age.
Booking appointment	Give proper information and advice about the risk of diabetes on pregnancy, birth and lactation
16 weeks	Retinal assessment for women with diabetic retinopathy in the first appointment.

20 weeks	Offer 4-chamber view of the fetal heart & outflow tracts (offer routine 18–20 weeks scan)
25 weeks	Routine antenatal care visit for nullipara
28 weeks	Offer ultrasound monitoring of fetal growth and amniotic fluid volume every 4 weeks Retinal assessment for women with no diabetic retinopathy in the first appointment.
32 weeks*	Offer ultrasound monitoring of fetal growth and amniotic fluid volume Offer routine antenatal care to nullipara
34 weeks	Routine antenatal care visit
36 weeks	Offer ultrasound monitoring of fetal growth and amniotic fluid volume

Discuss

- Timing and management of birth including analgesia and anaesthesia (anaesthetic assessment of women with diabetic complications e.g. obesity or autonomic neuropathy).
- Modification of hypoglycaemic therapy during and after birth
- Initial care of the newborn
- Initiation of breastfeeding, the effect of breastfeeding on glycaemic control
- Contraception and postpartum follow-up.

38 weeks	Offer labour induction versus Cesarean section (if indicated) Offer tests of fetal well-being if a woman wants to wait for spontaneous delivery.
39 weeks	Offer tests of fetal well-being if a woman wants to wait for spontaneous delivery.
40 weeks	Offer tests of fetal well-being if a woman wants to wait for spontaneous delivery.
41 weeks	Offer tests of fetal well-being if a woman wants to wait for spontaneous delivery.

* This visit replaces the routine 31-week visit in low risk nullipara

Gestational Diabetes

| Antenatal care |

| Booking appointment |----| Identify high risk women |

- BMI above 30 kg/m^2.
- Previous macrosomic baby weighing 4.5 kg or above.
- Previous gestational diabetes.
- First-degree relative with diabetes.
- Family origin with a high prevalence of diabetes (South Asian, black Caribbean and Middle Eastern).

| If there is previous diabetes | | If there is other risk factors |

| At 16-18 weeks | | At 24-28 weeks |

2-hour 75 g oral glucose tolerance test (OGTT)*   2-hour 75 g oral glucose tolerance test (OGTT)

If normal

Repeat at 28 weeks

If diagnosed

| Management of diabetes |

- Inform the woman that there is a small risk of complications during pregnancy if gestational diabetes is not controlled.
- Set up an individualized glucose target and advise self monitoring of blood glucose

| Initial treatment |

Diet, body weight and exercise
Most cases respond to this line of treatment. Weight loss is advised in women with a BMI > 27 ka/m^2

IF

No response to life style management within 1-2 weeks
OR
There is fetal macrosomia (abdominal circumference above the 70th percentile)

| Hypoglycemic treatment |

Regular insulin, the rapid acting insulin (aspart and lispro) and/or the oral hypoglycaemics (metformin and glibenclamide) may be considered.

Oral glucose tolerance test (OGTT)		WHO/NICE cutoff points	IADPSG*
	Fasting	≥ 7.0 mmol/l	≥ 5.1 mmol/l
	1 hour postprandial	-	≥ 10.0 mmol/l
	2 hour postprandial	≥ 7.8 mmol/l	≥ 8.5 mmol/l

* IADPSG = International Association of Diabetes and Pregnancy Study Groups

Intrapartum care

Counseling before labour

Discuss the mode of delivery including vaginal birth, labour induction and Cesarean section taking in consideration

The general indications of Cesarean section and ultrasonographic diagnosis of macrosomia.

The possibility of vaginal birth after previous Cesarean section or in the presence of diabetic retinopathy should be discussed.

Timing of delivery

Preterm labour

Reaches 38 weeks

Tocolytics

May be considered to stop premature contractions. However, beta-mimetic drugs are contraindicated.

Antenatal steroids

Given to enhance lung maturity. Consider close glucose monitoring and supplementary insulin dose according to an arranged protocol

Consider delivery either by Cesarean section or labour induction (consider Cesarean section indications, diabetic retinopathy and the presence of macrosomia before counseling)

Labour management

Assess blood glucose

Every 1 hour during labour

Every 30 minutes with general anaesthesia

The target is to maintain glucose between 4-7 mmol/L

If this level cannot be maintained or the woman has type 1 Diabetes

Consider intravenous dextrose and insulin

Blood glucose	IV fluids	Insulin
60-90 mg/dl	5% Glucose solution - 100 ml/hr	-
90-120 mg/dl	NS or RL* - 100 ml/hr	-
120-140 mg/dl	NS or RL - 100 ml/hr	4 units of Regular insulin
140-180 mg/dl	NS or RL - 100 ml/hr	6 units of Regular insulin
>180 mg/dl	NS or RL - 100 ml/hr	8 units of Regular insulin

* NS = normal saline. RL = Ringer's lactate

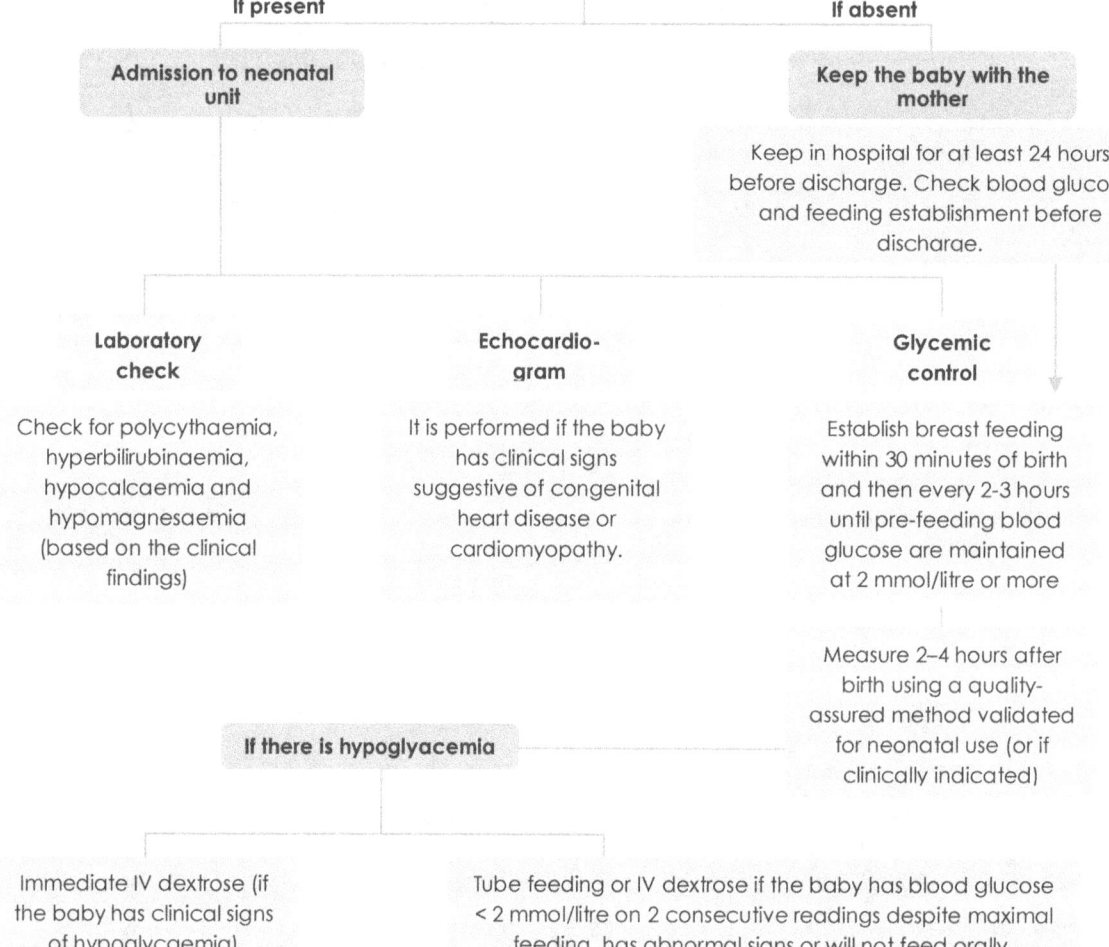

Neonatal care

Immediate assessment after birth

- The newborn is hypoglycaemic (abnormal signs)
- The newborn has respiratory distress or jaundice
- The newborn has cardiac decompensation, neonatal encephalopathy or polycythaemia
- The newborn needs intravenous fluids
- The newborn needs tube feeding (if not available on the postnatal ward)
- Preterm labour (before 34 weeks or between 34-36 weeks if dictated clinically).

If present   If absent

Admission to neonatal unit   **Keep the baby with the mother**

Keep in hospital for at least 24 hours before discharge. Check blood glucose and feeding establishment before discharge.

Laboratory check   **Echocardio-gram**   **Glycemic control**

Check for polycythaemia, hyperbilirubinaemia, hypocalcaemia and hypomagnesaemia (based on the clinical findings)

It is performed if the baby has clinical signs suggestive of congenital heart disease or cardiomyopathy.

Establish breast feeding within 30 minutes of birth and then every 2-3 hours until pre-feeding blood glucose are maintained at 2 mmol/litre or more

Measure 2–4 hours after birth using a quality-assured method validated for neonatal use (or if clinically indicated)

If there is hypoglyacemia

Immediate IV dextrose (if the baby has clinical signs of hypoglycaemia)

Tube feeding or IV dextrose if the baby has blood glucose < 2 mmol/litre on 2 consecutive readings despite maximal feeding, has abnormal signs or will not feed orally.

Postnatal care

Immediate counseling

- Women with diabetes who are breastfeeding should avoid unsafe drugs.
- Counsel her for contraception and pre-conception care in future pregnancies.

Treatment adjustment

Pre-existing diabetes

Gestational diabetes

Stop hypoglycemic medications immediately after birth
Advice on diet control, weight adjustment and exercise and inform about the symptoms of hyperglycemia

Assess blood glucose level before discharge.
Advise a fasting plasma glucose test at the 6-week postnatal appointment then every year.

Type 1 Diabetes (or type 2 on insulin)

Type 2 Diabetes Mellitus

Reduce insulin immediately after birth and self monitor glucose level to adjust the dose. Advise on the risk of hypoglycemia, there should be diet available before or during breastfeeding

Resume or continue using metformin and glibenclamide while breastfeeding. Other oral hypoglycemics are contraindicated

Return back to routine diabetes care after discharge.
Offer follow up for women with preproliferative diabetic retinopathy for at least 6 months after the birth.

| Appendix | **Fetal complications of diabetes with pregnancy** |

Fetal risks

Miscarriage

This risk is associated with pregestational diabetes rather than gestational diabetes which develops later in pregnancy. The risk is related to long standing diabetes with associated vasculopathy.

Congenital anomalies

There is 2-5 times increase in the risk of fetal anomalies (pregestational diabetes)
- Neural tube defects
- Cardiac anomalies (transposition of the great vessels)
- Renal anomalies
- Sacral agenesis (caudal regression syndrome): pathognomonic for diabetes

The risk of aneuploidy is not increased. However, it may be associated with lower MSAFP, beta HCG and E3.

Fetal macrosomia

The risk of feta macrosomia is 40-50% and is significantly related to glycaemic control. Maternal glucose (but not insulin) crosses the placenta and causes fetal hyperglycemia. This stimulates fetal pancreatic beta cells to secrete insulin which has an anabolic effect on the fetus. Growth is asymmetric affecting mainly the shoulder and trunk

- Increased risk of Cesarean section

- Increased risk of shoulder dystocia and birth trauma

- Risk of antenatal hypoxia and acidosis

IUGR

This is less common than fetal macrosomia. It is associated with maternal vasculopathy, hypertension and superimposed pre-eclampsia or nephropathy

Hydramnios

Polyhydramnios is a common finding in diabetes and is related to fetal polyuria

Prematurity

It is most commonly iatrogenic (due to IUGR, renal impairment or superimposed pre-eclampsia) but it occurs spontaneously in about 20% of cases especially in the presence of hydramnios

Fetal hypoxia

Fetal hypoxia and acidosis are associated with:
- Hyperglycemia and hyperinsulinaemia with lactic acid production
- Maternal vascular diseases

Stillbirth

There is an increased risk of stillbirth (5 times)

Neonatal risks

Neonatal hypoglyacemia

Fetal beta cell hyperplasia and neonatal hyperinsulinaemia causes hypoglycemia after maternal glucose is eliminated

Respiratory distress syndrome

The mechanism beyond the syndrome in women with diabetes is not fully understood

Others

Hypocalcaemia, hypomagnesaemia, polycythaemia and neonatal jaundice

STATION 5: MEDICAL DISORDERS WITH PREGNANCY

Obstetric Cholestasis

BACKGROUND   *What obstetrician should know about Obstetric Cholestasis*

Definitions

Obstetric cholestasis is a multifactorial disorder of pregnancy that is characterised by pruritus without skin rash and abnormal liver function tests (LFTs) which resolve after birth (in absence of other causes).

Prevalence

The prevalence is affected by genetic and environmental factors:
In England, the prevalence is generally 0.7%, reaching 1.2–1.5% in women of Indian–Asian or Pakistani–Asian origin.

Complications

- **Stillbirth:** the additional risk of stillbirth is not determined but is most likely to be small above the general population. The perinatal mortality rate from obstetric cholestasis is 5.7 to 11/1000
- **Prematurity:** the incidence of premature birth, especially iatrogenic (7-25%), is increased. Spontaneous preterm labour is slightly higher than the general population (4-12%).
- **Passage of meconium:** there is increased incidence of passage of meconium and fetal distress. Passage of meconium is more common in:
  - Preterm obstetric cholestasis (25%) than term obstetric cholestasis pregnancies (12%).
  - Severe obstetric cholestasis (bile acids over 40 micromoles/litre) than mild cholestasis (bile acids under 20 micromoles/litre).
- **Cesarean section:** Caesarean section rates are higher (10% to 36%).
- **Postpartum haemorrhage:** there is no evidence to support this association. The rate in available studies is 2-22%.

APPROACH   *How obstetricians should deal with Obstetric Cholestasis*

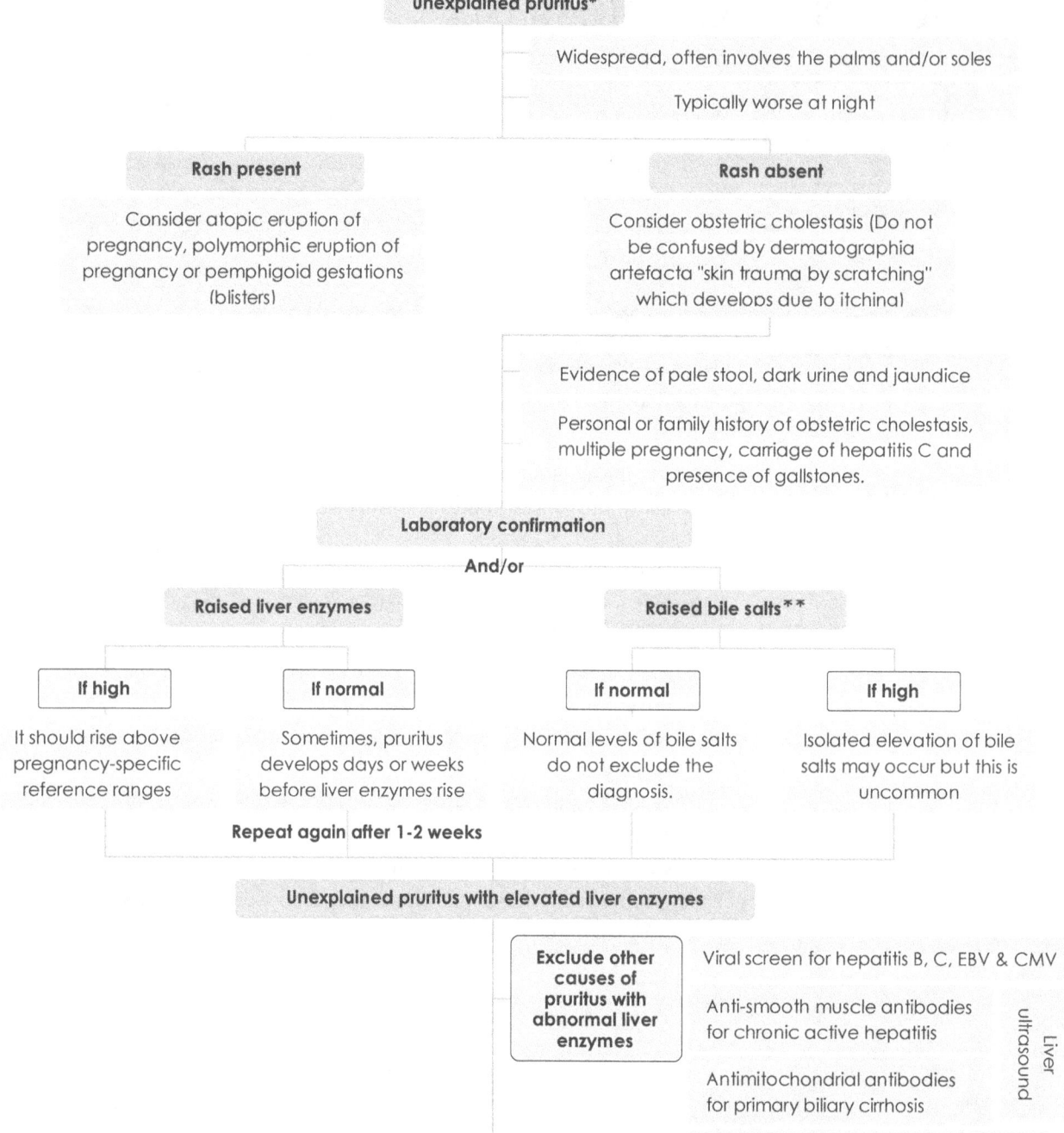

Unexplained pruritus*

Widespread, often involves the palms and/or soles

Typically worse at night

Rash present

Consider atopic eruption of pregnancy, polymorphic eruption of pregnancy or pemphigoid gestations (blisters)

Rash absent

Consider obstetric cholestasis (Do not be confused by dermatographia artefacta "skin trauma by scratching" which develops due to itching)

Evidence of pale stool, dark urine and jaundice

Personal or family history of obstetric cholestasis, multiple pregnancy, carriage of hepatitis C and presence of gallstones.

Laboratory confirmation

And/or

Raised liver enzymes

Raised bile salts**

If high

It should rise above pregnancy-specific reference ranges

If normal

Sometimes, pruritus develops days or weeks before liver enzymes rise

If normal

Normal levels of bile salts do not exclude the diagnosis.

If high

Isolated elevation of bile salts may occur but this is uncommon

Repeat again after 1-2 weeks

Unexplained pruritus with elevated liver enzymes

Exclude other causes of pruritus with abnormal liver enzymes

Viral screen for hepatitis B, C, EBV & CMV

Anti-smooth muscle antibodies for chronic active hepatitis

Antimitochondrial antibodies for primary biliary cirrhosis

Pre-eclampsia and acute fatty liver of pregnancy (early stages)

Liver ultrasound

Diagnosis of obstetric cholestasis

Initial diagnosis is to be confirmed postnatal by disappearance of pruritus and abnormal liver enzymes

* Pruritus: Pruritus in pregnancy affects 23% of pregnancies. Small proportion is due to obstetric cholestasis.

** Pregnancy specific bile salt levels should not be assumed. Bile acid level increases with meal and decreases with fasting and random levels are usually used

*** 20% lower than the non-pregnant range

Diagnosis of obstetric cholestasis

Consultant-led, team based care

Treatment

Follow up

Systemic

S-adenosvl methionine

It is not recommended

Ursodeoxvcholic acid

It improves pruritus and liver function

Dexamethasone

Not a first line.

Vitamin K

If PT** is prolonged

Topical

Topical emollients e.g. calamine lotion, aqueous cream with menthol are safe but the efficacy is unknown

Maternal

BP/urine check

For exclusion of other possible diagnoses of the clinical presentation

Liver enzymes weekly

If they increase rapidly or if they return to normal, the diagnosis should be revised

Fetal

Poor fetal outcome cannot be predicted by biochemical testing. There is no facility to predict fetal death including Ultrasound, cardiotocography and Doppler *

After 37 week of gestation

Counsel for delivery

Induction of labour

There is an increased risk of maternal and perinatal mortality***. However, it is strongly indicated with severe biochemical abnormality

Continue beyond 37 weeks

A woman should be advised that there is no method to predict stillbirth if she decides to continue pregnancy

Delivery in hospital unit

Continuous fetal monitoring should be offered

Postpartum care

Follow up

A health care practitioner should confirm that liver function tests return to normal, all abnormal investigations are normalized and pruritus is relieved

Liver function tests are not carried out in the first 10 days (liver enzymes normally increase in this period). It should be performed before the postnatal care visit (LFTs at 6 weeks, postnatal care visit at 8 weeks)

Counseling

There is no long-term sequence on the mother or the newborn

There is hiah recurrence rate (45-90%)

There is higher risk in family members

Counsel for contraception (estrogen containina methods should be avoided)

---

* Fetal death is usually sudden and is not an outcome of placental insufficiency, fetal growth restriction or oligohydramnios.

** PT = Prothrombin time

*** The risk of admission to a neonatal care unit after elective caesarean section is 7–11% at 37 weeks of gestation, 6% at 38 weeks of gestation and 1.5% at 39 weeks of gestation.

| Appendix | **Drug index for treatment of obstetric cholestasis** |

Colestyramine	A bile acid-chelating agent. It improves pruritus in some women but may also exacerbate vitamin K deficiency (risk of fetal intracranial haemorrhage). It is not of clinical use
Activated charcoal and guar gum	They do not relieve pruritus.
S-adenosyl methionine	There is no evidence to support its rule for maternal or fetal indications. It is not recommended
Ursodeoxycholic acid	• **Mechanism:** The mechanism of action is displacement of more hydrophobic endogenous bile salts from the bile acid. This protects the hepatocyte membrane from the damaging effect of bile salts and enhance bile acid clearance from the fetus. • **Action:** it improves pruritus and liver function. However, there is lack of evidence that it protects against stillbirth.
Dexamethasone	Dexamethasone (10 mg orally for 7 days and then stopping over 3 days) is not recommended as a first line therapy. It may cause some improvement of symptoms and biochemistry in some women. It should be given after thorough consultation.
Vitamin K	Vitamin K is given after maternal counseling: • It is advised whenever prothrombin time is prolonged, water-soluble vitamin K (menadiol sodium phosphate) in doses of 5–10 mg daily is given. • If prothrombin time is normal, low doses of water-soluble vitamin K may be given after careful counseling which includes discussion of benefits and the small risks. Women who take antiepileptic medications (at risk of vitamin K deficiency) show greater levels of vitamin K in the offspring if taking oral supplements before delivery compared with the offspring of those who did not.

STATION 5: MEDICAL DISORDERS WITH PREGNANCY

Epilepsy With Pregnancy

BACKGROUND *What obstetrician should know about epilepsy with pregnancy*

Effect of epilepsy on pregnancy

- **Infertility:** the probability of having children in both males and females is less than in general population. It is less than 50% in females with epilepsy. The possible causes are:
  - *Psychological factor:* these women are usually worried about having children and are particularly concerned about congenital anomalies.
  - *Reproductive endocrine disorders:* that may be associated with epilepsy e.g. polycystic ovarian syndrome and hypogonadotropic or hypergonadotropic hypogonadism.
  - *Anovulation:* anovulatory menstrual disturbance is more common in temporal lobe epilepsy than in normal women (35% versus 10%).
- **Fetal and neonatal complications:**
  - *Perinatal mortality:* the risk is twice that of normal population.
  - *Teratogenicity:* 2-3 fold increase in risk of congenital anomalies with anti-epileptic drugs. The risk depends on the following factors:
    - ◆ The dose (dose-related).
    - ◆ The number (the risk is more in women taking more than one drug/polytherapy – 15% versus 6.5%).
    - ◆ The timing (first trimester exposure carries the highest risk).
    - ◆ The drug (multiple drugs including valproate carry higher risk).
  - *Neonatal withdrawal:*
    Drug withdrawal e.g. jitteriness, hypotonia, hypoglycaemia, apnoeic episodes or seizures
- **Childhood complications:**
  - An increased incidence of neurodevelopmental delay in the first 2 years is suggested.
  - There is 4-5% risk of epilepsy among children, 10% if one affected sibling and 15-20% if both parents are affected (~1% general population).

Effect of pregnancy on epilepsy

The woman should be informed that the course of epilepsy during pregnancy is unpredictable . The severity of epilepsy may increase, decrease or remain stationary. Aggravation of epilepsy may be attributed to:
- Stress and fatigue during pregnancy.
- Non-compliance to therapy (for fear of teratogenesis).
- Decreased plasma drug level due to decreased absorption, vomiting, increased renal/hepatic clearance and decreased plasma albumin concentrations

APPROACH   *How obstetricians should deal with epilepsy with pregnancy*

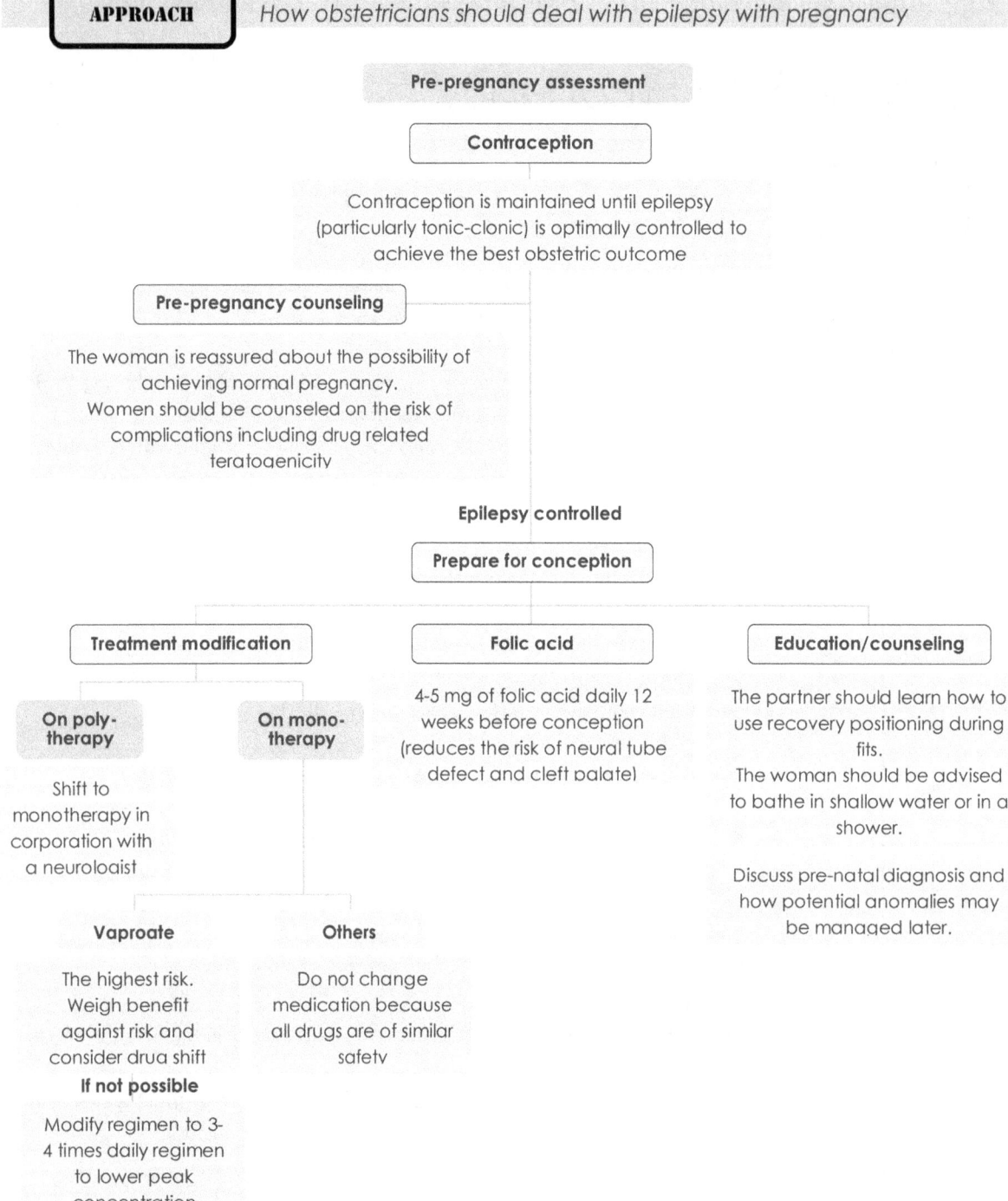

Pre-pregnancy assessment

Contraception

Contraception is maintained until epilepsy (particularly tonic-clonic) is optimally controlled to achieve the best obstetric outcome

Pre-pregnancy counseling

The woman is reassured about the possibility of achieving normal pregnancy.
Women should be counseled on the risk of complications including drug related teratogenicity

Epilepsy controlled

Prepare for conception

Treatment modification

Folic acid

4-5 mg of folic acid daily 12 weeks before conception (reduces the risk of neural tube defect and cleft palate)

Education/counseling

The partner should learn how to use recovery positioning during fits.
The woman should be advised to bathe in shallow water or in a shower.

Discuss pre-natal diagnosis and how potential anomalies may be managed later.

On poly-therapy

Shift to monotherapy in corporation with a neurologist

On mono-therapy

Vaproate

The highest risk. Weigh benefit against risk and consider drug shift
If not possible

Modify regimen to 3-4 times daily regimen to lower peak concentration

Others

Do not change medication because all drugs are of similar safety

If seizures are well controlled or if tonic-clonic seizures have not occurred, medication may be stopped during the first trimester or even during the entire pregnancy.

Antenatal care

First contact	Arrange for consultant-led care. A neurologist should be kept in contact if epilepsy is not well controlled. Advise that sleep deprivation may precipitate fits.	
First appointment	**Assessment**	Full history and clinical evaluation is performed
	Counseling	Risks and constitution of antenatal care should be discussed
	Screening	Offer routine screening for aneuploidy
	Monitoring	Monitor drug level in uncontrolled women (6-10 weeks)*
	Folic acid	Treatment should be continued during the first trimester
13 weeks	Re-continue drugs that may be stopped before conception after the first trimester	
15-16 weeks	Monitor drug level in uncontrolled women	
18-21 weeks	Offer general anomaly screening and fetal echocardiography	
28 weeks	Monitor drug level in uncontrolled women	
34-36 weeks	**Monitoring**	Monitor drug level in uncontrolled women
	Vitamin K	Reduces the risk of maternal/neonatal bleeding (oral, IM)
	Steroids	If indicated to enhance lung maturity, increase the dose of steroids if the woman is on liver enzyme inducing drugs

Labour

Arrange for delivery in a unit with specialized care including neonatal intensive care

Consider that epilepsy itself is not an indication for Cesarean section. However, the risk of epilepsy is highest during the peripartum period

Consider anti-epileptic drugs during labour

Non-oral treatment (IV or rectal) may be considered instead of oral treatment

Neonatal care

Examine the newborn for congenital anomalies. Give IM vitamin K to minimize the risk of haemorrhage (maximum in the first day)

---

* The rationale of drug monitoring is to optimize drug dose in uncontrolled women. The level of anti-epileptic drugs change during pregnancy e.g. maximum decline in phenytoin and phenobarbital levels occur during the first trimester, during the third trimester for carbamazepine. Valproate levels continue to fall during pregnancy.

Postpartum care

Continue pre-pregnancy regimen

Breast-feeding

The concentration of antiepileptic drugs in breast milk is determined by plasma level and protein binding

Phenytoin and valproic acid

Phenytoin in breast milk is present in only 18% of maternal circulation. Valproic acid in breast milk is 5% of maternal circulation. So they are appropriate for breast feeding (high protein binding)

lamotrigine and gabapentin

Information is lacking

Carbamazepine and phenobarbital

Carbamazepine in breast milk is 40% of maternal circulation level and phenobarbital is 36% of maternal level. However, They are still appropriate of breast feeding

Contraception

Women on anti-epileptic drugs that do not induce hepatic enzyme *

No impact on hormonal contraceptives.

Women on anti-epileptic drugs that induce hepatic enzyme **

Oral combined contraceptives: higher dose is required (50 µg). Low dose oral contraceptives (35 µg) are associated with high failure rate (6%).

Mini-pills: their efficacy is reduced.

Depo-provera: no need to increase the dose.

* Anti-epileptics that do not induce the P-450 system: Benzodiazepines, gabapentin, lamotrigine, valproate
** Anti-epileptics that induce hepatic enzymes (carbamazepine, phenytoin, primidone, topiramate)

Appendix ▌ **Safety profile of anti-epileptic drugs during pregnancy**

Phenytoin

- Fetal hydantion syndrome (fetal anti-epileptic drug syndrome):
  - *Major malformations:*
    - Heart defects.
    - Cleft lip or palate.
    - Skeletal malformations.
    - microcephaly.
  - *Minor malformations:*
    - Strabismus.
    - Hypertelorism.
    - Distal digital and nail hypoplasia.
    - Clubfoot.
    - Abnormal dermatoglyphic patterns.
- **Coagulopathy:** occurs in ~50% of babies born to mothers (vitamin K dependent clotting factor deficiency). However, very few of these babies are symptomatic.

Phenobarbital

- **Minor anomalies:** as with phenytoin.
- **Neonatal effects:** Exposed infants can have barbiturate depression or drug withdrawal at birth

Carbamazepine

Neural tube defects (NTD): 1% versus 0.1% in the general population. If the drug is given after the period of neural tube closure (days 22-29), there is no risk of NTD.

Valproic acid

Neural tube defects (spina pifida): 1-2% versus 0.1% in the general population. Infants exposed to more than 1,000 mg/day are at higher risk.

Gabapentin

Delayed bone ossification and hydronephrosis: in animal studies.

Generally, the risk of congenital anomalies is 6.5% with exposure to one drug, 15% with exposure to polytherapy.

STATION 5: MEDICAL DISORDERS WITH PREGNANCY

Chronic renal disease with pregnancy

BACKGROUND   *What obstetrician should know about chronic renal disease in pregnancy*

Incidence   The incidence varies from 2-12 per 10 000 women. Pregnancy is generally not expected in women with chronic renal disease.

Obstetric changes

- **Anatomic changes:** there is increase in kidney size and dilation of pelvicalyceal system.
- **Physiologic changes:**
  - *Renal plasma flow:* increases in the first trimester, reaches the maximum in the second trimester and then falls to about 50% above non-pregnancy level in the third trimester.
  - *The glomerular filtration rate (GFR):* increases significantly and serum creatinine and urea fall. Proteinuria should not exceed 300 mg/24 hours. However, in chronic renal diseases, the rise in GFR may be subnormal or it may even decrease. This may depend on the GFR itself and the presence significant proteinuria (> 1g/dl) rather than the presence of hypertension or underlying kidney disease.

| APPROACH | *How obstetricians should deal with chronic renal disease in pregnancy* |

Pre-pregnancy assessment

Counseling

Multidisciplinary team (MDT) Counseling

Counseling for conception

Counsel about the risk of pre-eclampsia, fetal growth restriction and preterm delivery. Counsel about the long-term deterioration in renal function after pregnancy.

If prepregnancy renal function is normal or mildly impaired (serum creatinine below 125 µmol/l (1.4 mg/dl)

Reassure the patient that obstetric progress will most likely be successful without impact on her renal function. However, complications including pre-eclampsia are still liable to occur

Counseling for infertility

Consider infertility work up and assessment of renal condition. If IVF is indicated for management, Single embryo transfer is recommended.

Medical modification

Blood pressure should be controlled. Angiotensin-converting enzyme (ACE) inhibitors and angiotensin receptor blockers protect renal function. They are recommended prior to pregnancy. Shift to safe drugs is advised after the woman becomes pregnant.

Consider women on immunosuppressive drugs

Do not discontinue prednisolone, azathioprine, ciclosporin or tacrolimus alone or in combination (not associated with fetal abnormalities).

Mycophenolate mofetil/enteric-coated mycophenolic acid, sirolimus/everolimus or rituximab are controversial. Their potential risks have not yet been determined

Antenatal care

Multidisciplinary team care

Multidisciplinary team care includes midwives, a maternal medicine specialist and a nephrologist. This is recommended to be carried out in a tertiary center

Obstetric care

First appointment

Low dose aspirin

For pre-eclampsia prophylaxis (from the 12th week)

Renal biopsy?[1]

Consider nephrotic syndrome

Early ultrasound scan

For accurate estimation of gestational age

Thrombo-prophylaxis [2]

Anomaly scan

The same approach like in normal pregnancy taking into account the unreliability of serum screening. Urinary tract should be screened in detail to exclude inherited conditions such as obstructive uropathy.

Frequent antenatal visits

Hypertension detected

Maintain blood pressure > 140/90 [4] using methyldopa, calcium channel blockers, hydralazine and labetalol

ve+ urinary screening

Bacterial vaginosis, urinary tract infections, asymptomatic bacteriuria should be managed to reduce the risk of prematurity

3rd trimester close care

Regular scans are carried out every 4 weeks from 28 weeks onwards. This is done to check fetal growth and amniotic fluid volume.

Basic investigations

Request as early as possible in pregnancy:
- **A baseline renal profile:** serum urea, creatinine, electrolytes, albumin and full blood count.
- **Urinalysis and urine culture:** are indicated.
- **Assessment of proteinuria[3]:** either by using a 24-hour collection of urine or by a spot test for total urine protein: creatinine ratio "PCR" (recommended, time saving). PCR is used for follow up.

Repeat at least every 4 weeks

If anaemia is diagnosed

Hct > 19%

Oral/intravenous iron therapy

Hct < 19%

Add recombinant erythropoietin

If hypertension develops or becomes aggravated

Use blood transfusion instead

If dialysis is indicated

If there is

- Severe refractory metabolic acidosis
- Severe refractory hyperkalemia
- Volume overload causing congestive heart failure
- Pulmonary oedema unresponsive to diuretics

Carry out renal dialysis even early in pregnancy for the risk of fetal demise

Nephrologist referral

Persistent proteinuria above 500 mg /day before 20 weeks

---

1 Renal biopsy in pregnancy may be indicated in florid nephrotic syndrome early in pregnancy or suspected rapidly progressive glomerulo-nephritis.

2 Women with nephrotic syndrome should receive prophylactic heparin in pregnancy as well as for 6 weeks

3 If dipstick test for proteinuria is +1 or more (infection excluded), proteinuria should be quantified.

4 Tight versus non-tight control is controversial because there is a concept that every 10 mm fall in mean arterial pressure is associated with a 145 g reduction in mean birth weight.

Intra-natal care

- pre-eclampsia
- Fetal growth restriction
- Rapidly deteriorating maternal renal function.
- Fetal deterioration

Yes

Early delivery planned

No

Delivery at or near term

Vaginal delivery	**Cesarean section**
The classic route	Based on obstetrics indications

Postnatal care

Microscopic haematuria in an otherwise normal kidney during pregnancy is investigated postpartum

Evaluation

Women with early onset pre-eclampsia (less than 32 weeks) are evaluated for an underlying renal cause

Postnatal combined clinic follow up
Combined obstetric and nephrology team care

Counseling for contraception
Should be established before discharge

Continue anticoagulant therapy
For 6 weeks postpartum in women with nephrotic syndrome

Pregnancy after renal transplantation

Pre-pregnancy counseling

- **Acute rejection:** counsel on the risk of pregnancy on acute rejection and graft loss. The risk correlates with:
  1. The pre-pregnancy serum creatinine levels
  2. The interval between transplant and pregnancy.

  The incidence of acute rejection is 9-14% (5% for serious episodes).
- **Chronic rejection:** the risk is not yet known.
- **Long-term survival of the graft:** counsel on the long-term survival of the graft. It is similar in pregnancy and non pregnant women.

Decide pregnancy if
- No rejection in the previous year
- Graft function is adequate and stable
- No or minimal proteinuria (<500 mg/24 hours)
- Woman on maintenance immunosuppression with stable dosage
- No acute infections that may harm the fetus (cytomegalovirus)
- Co-morbid conditions (hypertension, diabetes) are optimally managed

Screening for infection
Screen for cytomegalovirus (recheck titre in each trimester if negative), HIV, herpes simplex virus and hepatitis B and C.

Screening — Antenatal care — Management

Screening for gestational diabetes
Screening by oral glucose tolerance tests or blood sugar monitoring (if strongly suspicious)

Management of hypertension

- **Alpha methyldopa, labetalol and nifedipine:** are safe.
- **Magnesium sulphate prophylaxis:** in severe preeclampsia is also safe.
  - The loading dose is the same.
  - The infusion of magnesium is decreased (according to the level of elevated creatinine over the normal pregnancy level).

Uric acid is a not a significant marker in these patients (it may be raised even without pre-eclampsia).

Immunosuppressive therapy

- **Continue immunosuppressive drugs:** with the same prepregnancy dose.
- **Prednisolone, azathioprine, ciclosporin and tacrolimus:** are all safe
- **Mycophenolate mofetil ('MMF'):** is unsafe (increased risk of malformations and first-trimester pregnancy loss).

  The most frequent malformations include external ear and other facial malformations such as cleft palate and lip.
- **Rituximab, sirolimus or everolimus:** little evidence about safety. They should be avoided.

  Breastfeeding while on immunosuppressive drugs is controversial because of concerns for the effects on the baby (not absolute).

Delivery at 38-40 weeks

Intrapartum care

Vaginal birth

The classic route. Both oxytocin and prostaglandins are safe

Consider neonatal thymic atrophy, transient Leucopenia/thrombocytopenia, adrenocortical insufficiency, septicaemia and cytomegalovirus/hepatitis infection.

Cesarean section

It is considered in obstetric indications. Involvement of urology or renal transplant surgeons is advisable in elective caesarean section. Consider stress dosage steroids in women who are on immune-suppressive dosages of steroids.

Appendix | **Pregnancy in women on dialysis**

| Incidence | Conception is more likely in women with residual renal function and those who begin dialysis. The incidence of pregnancy is lower in women on peritoneal dialysis than on haemodialysis. |

Obstetric complications	

- **Spontaneous miscarriage:** is common (21% of second trimester pregnancies).
- **Preterm delivery:** is common (the mean gestational age is 32 weeks).
- **Polyhydramnios:** in 42–79% of pregnancies.
- **Neonatal mortality (50-70%):**
  - Large proportion is due to prematurity.
  - Perinatal outcome is better for women who conceive prior to starting dialysis than those who conceive after dialysis (73.6% versus 40.2%).
  - There is no significant difference in infant survival between women who receive peritoneal dialysis and those who receive haemodialysis.
- **Maternal complications:**
  - Hypertension (40–80%), hypertensive crisis and pre-eclampsia
  - Anaemia.
  - Placental abruption.
  - High Cesarean section rate: about 50% of these women due to the above complications.

Management

| **General lines** |

- **Protein intake:** increase protein intake to:
  - 1.5 g/kg/day in women on haemodialysis.
  - 1.8 g/kg/day in women on peritoneal dialysis.
  Weight gain of 0.5 kg/week is expected.
- **Fluid intake:** is individualized on basis of:
  - Native urine output.
  - The type/frequency of renal replacement therapy the woman is receiving.
- **Calcium supplementation:** 1.5 g/day (calcium dialysate).
- **25-hydroxy vitamin D measurement:** in each trimester and supplementation if low.
- **Oral phosphate supplements:** if its level is low (it is usually high in women on dialysis).
- **Folate supplementation:** 5 mg/day for all women.
- **Multivitamin supplementation:** vitamin C, thiamine, riboflavin, niacin and vitamin B6 are given.

| **Haemodialysis** |

- **The frequency of dialysis:** it increases to at least 20 hours per week.
- **The aim is to:**
  1. Maintain a predialysis blood urea of 15–20 mmol/l.
  2. Avoid maternal volume depletion and hypotension (maintain diastolic pressure between 80-90 mmHg) during dialysis (smaller surface area dialyser to reduce the ultrafiltration rate per treatment is recommended).
  3. Adjust the amount of bicarbonate and potassium in the dialysate to avoid electrolyte imbalance due to frequent dialysis.

Management (cont.)

Peritoneal dialysis

- Peritoneal dialysis is safe during pregnancy with the following percussions:
  - Increase the number of exchanges during pregnancy.
  - Reduce the fill volumes of peritoneal dialysis fluid to 1–1.5 l.
  - Switch to haemodialysis when pregnancy becomes advanced (the enlarging uterus makes peritoneal dialysis inapplicable).
- If caesarean section: is indicated, the following percussions should be considered:
  - Perform it extraperitoneally or
  - Perform temporary haemodialysis postpartum following caesarean section.

Treatment of anaemia

- **Keep haemoglobin between 10–11 g/dl:** the erythropoietin dose should increase by 50–100%
- **Maintain iron saturation of 30% or more:** through IV iron supplementation.

STATION 5: MEDICAL DISORDERS WITH PREGNANCY

Urinary tract infection with pregnancy

| **BACKGROUND** | *What obstetrician should know about UTI with pregnancy* |

Definitions

The presence of 10^5 bacteria/ml in a mid-stream urine sample. This high number minimizes the possibility of bacterial contamination to less than 1% (50% if 103-4 is used). The diagnosis is confirmed by the isolation of only one uropathogen (or predominantly one) from culture.

A mid-stream urine sample can perfectly be obtained by suprapubic aspiration or by a sterile catheter sample. However, decontamination of urethral meatus is the most practical method of obtaining a less contaminated mid stream sample.

Incidence

The incidence of UTI during pregnancy is 8%:

*   The incidence of asymptomatic bacteriuria in pregnant women is 2–5%.
*   The incidence of acute cystitis is 1.3%.
*   The incidence of pyelonephritis during pregnancy is 2% (up to 23% experience recurrence).

Classification

Asymptomatic bacteriuria	Significant numbers of bacteria (10^5) in a mid-stream urine sample without urinary symptoms.
Acute cystitis	Significant numbers of bacteria along with lower urinary tract symptoms (dysuria, urgency, frequency, nocturia, haematuria, suprapubic discomfort) without fever or general manifestations.
Pyelonephritis	Significant numbers of bacteria along with upper urinary tract symptoms (flank or renal angle pain) and systemic manifestations (fever, rigors, nausea and vomiting).

Aetiology

Risk factors	**Organisms**

• **Generally:** women have short urethra. Intercourse also traumatizes the distal urethra allowing easy bacterial invasion.
 • **During pregnancy:**
  ▪ *Anatomically:* Bladder volume increases and detrusor activity decreases, the ureter dilates under the relaxing effect of progesterone and uterine pressure (right).
  ▪ *Chemically:* Glucosuria is present in 70% of pregnant women. Aminoaciduria is present. Urine osmolality drops.
  ▪ *Immunologically:* theoretically, pregnant women are immunologically deficient facilitating bacterial invasion.
	Like non pregnant, E-coli is the commonest (80-90%). Staphylococcus Saprophyticus is the 2nd. Generally, GIT pathogens only can grow in urine. GBS Bacteriuria carries a risk of PROM - preterm labour

APPROACH   *How obstetricians should deal with UTI in pregnancy*

First   Women with asymptomatic bacteriuria

Early pregnancy screening

Screening for asymptomatic bacteriuria early in
pregnancy is grade A recommendation by the RCOG

Approach   Counseling

How to screen*   Why to screen

Single urine culture with
optimal technique (gold
standard despite the cost and   Consider maternal hazards   Consider fetal hazards
time needed for culture,
which extends between 24-   Symptomatic cystitis (30%)   Prematurity, low birth weight
48 hours).   Pyelonephritis (50%)   Fetal growth restriction
                                  Preterm labour and delivery   Stillbirth
                                  Preeclampsia,   Perinatal mortality
                        6%   Anaemia   Mental retardation and
Negative   Positive   Chorioamnionitis and   developmental delay.
                                  postpartum endometritis   (bacterial endotoxin effect
Consider treatment to   and cerebral hypoperfusion
reduce the risk of   are accused)
pyelonephritis, preterm
labour and low birth
weight

Urine culture
and sensitivity

Start
antibiotics

Continue for 7 days**

Follow up

Follow up by urine culture is indicated as long
as the diagnosis is established. Recurrence is
possible after treatment is completed. Follow
up continues till delivery.

* Simple urine-based screening methods like interleukin-8 test and rapid enzymatic test are far less specific and sensitive
than urine culture and cannot be considered for screening (RCOG recommendations)
** Evidence of shorter courses has not yet been established.

Second | **Women with acute cystitis (1%)**

Women with lower urinary tract symptoms without general illness

Consider clinical assessment

Urethral discharge? → Acute urethral syndromes

Associated vulvitis, vaginitis/cervicitis? → Secondary causes are suspicious e.g. Herpes

Dipstick detection of nitrite

Simple safe analgesics can be used (topical agents have no rule)

Increased fluid oral intake to dilute pathogens is not supported while awaiting culture results. This may exacerbate urinary symptoms.

Alkalinizing agents are not recommended (for hypernatremia, the risk of sodium citrate during pregnancy). They effectiveness is also doubtful.

If positive

Consider bacterial count

Start empirical antibiotic therapy

Urine culture and sensitivity

Significant bacteriuria

Modify antibiotic choice according to bacterial sensitivity results

Continue treatment for 7-10 days

No significant bacteriuria

Acute urethral syndromes*
(associated urethral discharge)

Failure or relapse

Start another antibiotic according to sensitivity for 7 days

Consider an underlying pathology

Follow the woman up

* Gonococcal and nongonococcal urethritis (Chlamydia) infections

Third — Women with pyelonephritis (2% - 2nd and 3rd trimester)

Pyelonephritis is serious. Untreated infection can end up with pyonephrosis, perinephric abscess, septicaemia and septic shock.

Women with fever, rigors, nausea, vomiting, pain and tenderness of renal angle, maternal and fetal tachycardia ± lower urinary tract symptoms

Mild presentation

Outpatient treatment with antibiotics (consider higher doses than non-pregnant requirements or hydrophilic drugs because of diluted plasma, increased elimination rate during pregnancy)

Severe presentation (usual)

Hospital admission

A full history and clinical examination
Assessment of fetal wellbeing
Blood culture (aerobic and anaerobic)
Vaginal swabs
Mid stream urine culture

Empirical antibiotic therapy initiated (after drawing samples for culture)
Begin with broad sectrum parentral antibiotics (e.g. cephalosporins)

Simple analgesia for renal pain (avoid NSAIDs*, consider paracetamol as a safe choice, renal colic may necessitate opioids)

Thromboprophylaxis (graduated compression stockings and low molecular weight heparin) if prolonged bed rest is needed

Tocolysis is commonly used because of preterm labour risk. If threatened preterm labour develops, consider antenatal steroids

Re-evaluate treatment regimen after 24-48 hours if there is no response
(a resistant organism is especially susceptible)

Culture results revealed

Re-evaluate your antibiotic choice accordingly

Lack of response

Consider an underlying renal pathology or renal anomaly

Other specialists should be involved (urologists, nephrologists and microbiologists). Radiological consultation is essential **

If severe sepsis/septic shock are suspicious

Start clinical evaluation, resuscitation and investigations immediately followed by Specialist consultation and ICU admission

Good response

Continue antibiotic treatment for at least 10 days (and up to 2-3 weeks to minimize relapse). Fever should be absent for at least 24 hours. Urine should turn sterile

---

* NSAIDs carry maternal risks e.g. renal effects and fetal risks e.g. premature closure of ductus arteriosus, oligohydramnios
** For recurrent cases, long-term low dose antibiotics can be considered till delivery or single postcoital treatment doses are given (because re-infection from the vagina following intercourse by coliform bacteria may occur).

STATION 5: MEDICAL DISORDERS WITH PREGNANCY

Thyroid disorders with pregnancy

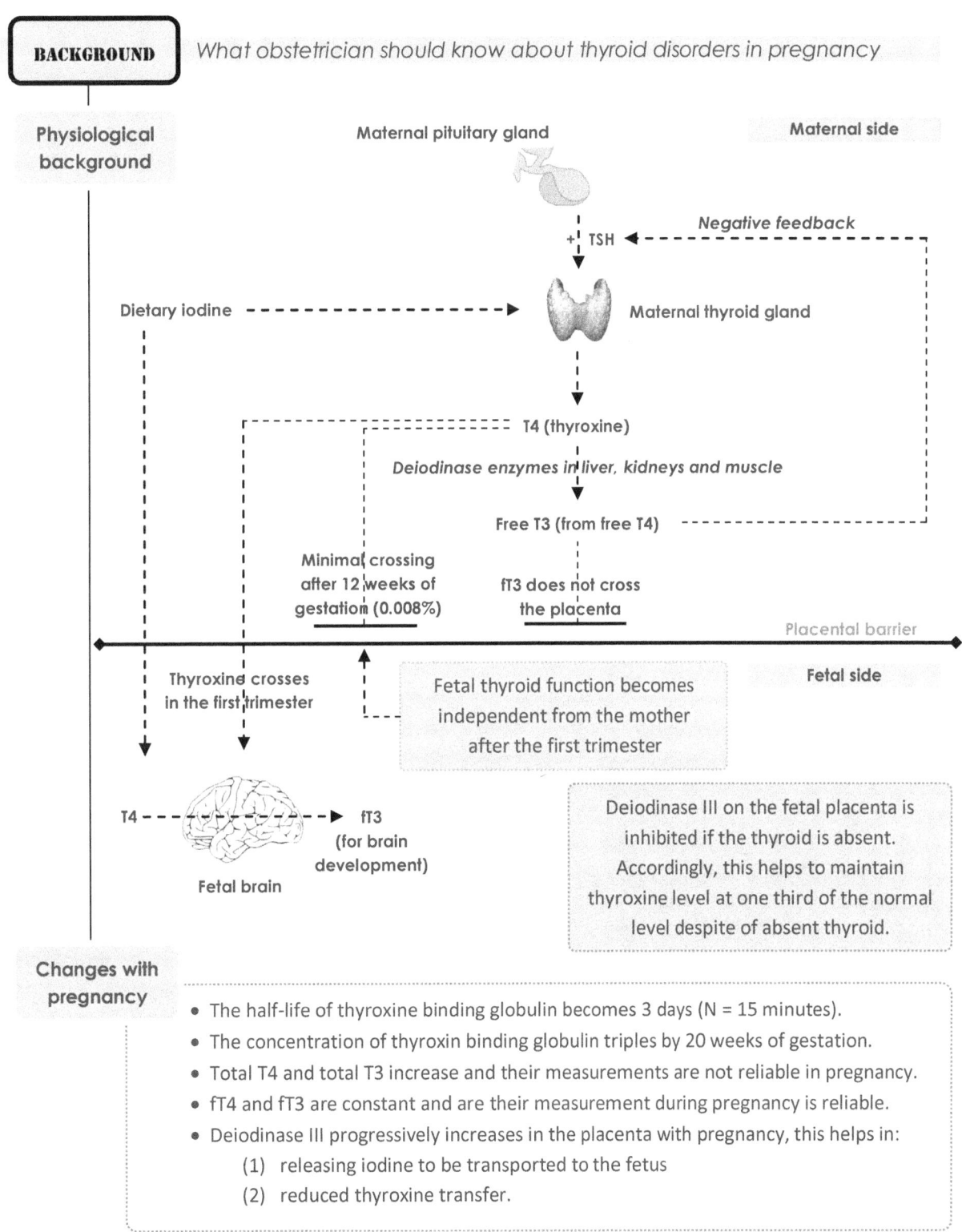

BACKGROUND   *What obstetrician should know about thyroid disorders in pregnancy*

Physiological background

Maternal pituitary gland   **Maternal side**

+ TSH ←--- *Negative feedback*

Dietary iodine ----→ Maternal thyroid gland

T4 (thyroxine)

Deiodinase enzymes in liver, kidneys and muscle

Free T3 (from free T4)

Minimal crossing after 12 weeks of gestation (0.008%)

fT3 does not cross the placenta

Placental barrier

Thyroxine crosses in the first trimester

Fetal thyroid function becomes independent from the mother after the first trimester

Fetal side

T4 ---→ fT3 (for brain development)

Fetal brain

Deiodinase III on the fetal placenta is inhibited if the thyroid is absent. Accordingly, this helps to maintain thyroxine level at one third of the normal level despite of absent thyroid.

Changes with pregnancy

- The half-life of thyroxine binding globulin becomes 3 days (N = 15 minutes).
- The concentration of thyroxin binding globulin triples by 20 weeks of gestation.
- Total T4 and total T3 increase and their measurements are not reliable in pregnancy.
- fT4 and fT3 are constant and are their measurement during pregnancy is reliable.
- Deiodinase III progressively increases in the placenta with pregnancy, this helps in:
    (1) releasing iodine to be transported to the fetus
    (2) reduced thyroxine transfer.

APPROACH   *How obstetricians should deal with thyroid disease in pregnancy*

First   Women with hypothyroidism (1%)

Pre-pregnancy assessment by thyroid function test

Adjustment of thyroxine dose prior to pregnancy

Early first trimester assessment by thyroid function test [1]

Adjustment of thyroxine dose is essential for fetal brain development [2]

Established case	Undiagnosed case	Established case
Normal fT4 and TSH?	Normal fT4, raised TSH	low fT4 and high TSH?
Optimal control	**Subclinical hypothyroidism**	**Suboptimal control**
Continue with the same dose of thyroxine and follow up	The use of thyroxine replacement in these women is debatable	Rapid adjustment of thyroxine dose (between 25-50 micrograms)

Adjustment of dose according to fT4 and TSH trimester specific ranges [3]

Continue antenatal care

Repeat thyroid function once at the second and third trimester. Thyroxine is adjusted for maternal rather than fetal causes [4]

Continue follow up through antenatal care. The majority of antenatal care can be carried out through midwives (unless complicated)

[1] Thyroid function test is the target of thyroxine dose adjustment and not the clinical presentation because both hypo and hyperthyroidism may be mistaken with normal pregnancy symptoms.
[2] A correlation has not been clearly proven
[3] To adjust according to TSH or fT4 is still questionable
[4] Hypothyroidism is not related to poor obstetric outcome

Second   Women with hyperthyroidism (Grave's = 0.2%)

Diagnosis of pregnancy

Clinically

Women with manifestations of hyperthyroidism (may be mistaken with pregnancy symptoms), most specifically:

- Failure to gain weight with good appetite.
- Tachycardia > 100 beats per minute (not reduced with the Valsalva manoeuvre).
- onycholysis.
- Eye signs and pretibial myxoedema (not related to disease activity).

Biochemically

- *Thyroid function test:* is measured in women known to have hyperthyroidism assessed in relation to trimester-specific reference ranges.
- *TSH receptor stimulating antibody titre:* this reflects disease activity (it rises in the first trimester and puerperium and falls in the second and third trimesters).

Control clinical symptoms

Beta blockers

They are targeted to control symptoms. Maternal and fetal advantages overweigh the risk of intrauterine growth restriction associated with these drugs

Block thyroid synthesis and lower antibody titre

Anti-thyroid drugs

Use the lowest effective dose to avoid fetal hypothyroidism. Propylthiouracil is preferred over carbimazole. Counsel the woman to report sore throats (risk of agranulocytosis)

Continue antenatal care

Maternal care

Fetal care

After 20 weeks, monitor the fetus for the signs of fetal thyrotoxicosis (fetal Graves') if the mother has Graves' or history of Graves' (monitor for tachycardia, excessive movements, fetal growth restriction, oligohydramnios and goitre)

If well controlled

Continue biochemical follow up monthly

If the patient has:

Compression by large goitre

Suspicion of malignancy

Failed antithyroid therapy

Consider surgery

If relapse or new diagnosis

Continue biochemical follow up more frequently

Surgery is considered by a skilled surgeon (the gland is highly vascular during pregnancy) usually in the 2nd trimester
Radioactive iodine is contraindicated

During labour

Cord blood sampling for thyroid function assessment

Neonatal hyperthyroidism is occasionally diagnosed due to transplacental passage of TSH receptor stimulating antibodies*

Repeat after 7-10 days because the half-life of antithyroid drugs is shorter than the half-life of these antibodies Consider clinical signs like poor feeding and weight loss

Neonatal hypothyroidism is rarely diagnosed due to transplacental passage of antithyroid drugs (self-limiting).

Management during puerperium

Neonatal

Maternal

If treatment is indicated, it is usually for few months

Medical treatment

High doses especially of carbimazole may cause neonatal hypothyroidism. So divide the dose throughout the day, breast feed before the next dose, monitor the newborn regularly and consider shifting to propylthiouracil

Radioactive iodine

Lactation should stop 4 weeks prior to treatment

* These antibodies are seen in Grave's disease even if the woman is previously treated with surgery or radioactive iodine

Fact Box: Thyroid problems with pregnancy

- In the first trimester, hCG stimulates TSH receptor due to biochemical similarity giving the clinical picture of hyperthyroidism (women with multiple pregnancy, trophoblastic disease and hyperemesis gravidarum because the concentration of hCG and the thyrotropic subtypes increase).
- The pregnant woman is liable to iodine deficiency because of:
  (1) Increased glomerular filtration.
  (2) Increased uptake of iodine by the thyroid gland
  (3) Transplacental transfer
- When there is severe maternal iodine deficiency, maternal iodine uptake represents a priority with subsequent cretinism.
- We do not have to change the dose of thyroxine in women with hypothyroidism based on the normal physiologic changes with pregnancy because:
  (1) Increased thyroxine binding proteins and total thyroid hormone pool do not indicate increased dose.
  (2) Deiodinase II (converts T4 to T3 in the brain) increases with advancing gestation, this compensated when fT4 is low.

Fact Box: Why may we need to adjust thyroxine during pregnancy?

Factors with influence the dose of thyroxine in pregnant women with hypothyroisism:

- **Decreased absorption:** due to nausea and vomiting in the first trimester.
- **Defective absorption:** due to thyroxine binding to iron and calcium supplements
- **Lack of proper control:** prior to conception.
- **Poor compliance:** due to improper counseling and concerns about the safety of these drugs during pregnancy.
- **Normal variation:** in thyroxine dose during pregnancy.

Fact Box: Management of hyperthyroidism

- Propylthiouracil is preferred over carbimazole because it is more protein pound (less placental transfer) and because of the rare risk of aplasia cutis congenita of infant scalp with carbimazole. However, both factors are found to be insignificant and the priority is to protect the fetus by proper control during the first trimester.
- Radioactive iodine is contraindicated during pregnancy because it can cross the placenta and destroy fetal thyroid.

Fact Box: Complications of uncontrolled hyperthyroidism

- **Maternal:**
  - Thyroid storm
  - Congestive heart failure
  - Pre-eclampsia
- **Fetal:**

  Women with Grave's disease rarely suffer complications with good control. The risk of TSH receptor antibodies start after 20 weeks of gestation when fetal thyroid can respond to these antibodies and the risk is proportional to the antibody titre (but still low even if the titre is high). These are possible the fetal risks:
  - Craniosynostosis and intellectual impairment
  - Hydrops fetalis
  - Prematurity
  - Intrauterine death
  - Polyhydramnios (due to oesophageal pressure).
  - Obstructed labour (neck extension related to goiter).
- **Neonatal:**
  - Neonatal hypothyroidism due to transplacental passage of antithyroid drugs (self-limiting).
  - Neonatal hyperthyroidism due to transplacental passage of TSH receptor stimulating antibodies

Appendix I | **In utero iodine deficiency**

Incidence

Iodine deficiency affects 2–10% of people in endemic areas and It causes mild mental handicap in 10–50%.

Pathophysiology

- In iodine deficiency, maternal T4 is depressed while maternal T3 level is kept normal. Accordingly, the mother will be compensated. However, T3 does not cross the placenta, and the fetal brain depends on maternal T4 to be transferred to the fetus and then to be converted to T3 to serve fetal brain development (early). T4 transfer will be inadequate even with inactivation of placenta deiodinase. Furthermore, even internal production of T4 by fetal thyroid later in pregnancy will be suppressed by deficiency of maternal iodine that crosses the placenta.
- The most affected structures of fetal brain (mostly in the second trimester) are the developing cochlea, cerebral neocortex and basal ganglia are most sensitive to iodine deficiency. This will cause:
  - Deaf-mutism.
  - Intellectual impairment.
  - Spastic motor disorder.
- Less severe maternal iodine deficiency causes only mental impairment (myxoedematous cretinism)

Diagnosis

- Low/very low T4
- Normal T3
- Raised TSH
- Compensatory goitre.

Management

Iodine administration prior to conception or up to the second trimester can prevent fetal sequences including miscarriage and pregnancy losses. However, there is no current strategy to supply iodine regularly to susceptible women.

Appendix II   **Hyperemesis gravidarum and thyroid problems**

Hyperemesis gravidarum

Thyroid function test

Conclusion of hyperthyroidism

Transient hyperthyroidism (60% of women with severe hyperemesis). This is caused by:

- TSH-like effect of the beta subunits of hCG.
- Increased total concentration of hCG (e.g. multiple pregnancy).
- Greater affinity of beta subunits of hCG to bind to TSH receptors.

Rare, first trimester Graves' disease that may be presented by severe vomiting. This diagnosis is serious and should not be missed

Differentiation

- Detailed history
- Normalization of thyroid biochemistry after hyperemesis resolves (maximum 19 weeks).
- No eye signs or goiter.
- Tachycardia responds to intravenous rehydration.

In case of doubt

Absence of thyroid autoantibodies supports the diagnosis of hyperemesis. However, the presence of antibodies does not exclude the diagnosis.

hCG-related thyrotoxicosis does not require anti-thyroid treatment, these medications are usually useless or may require very high doses to give response. High doses may cause fetal hypothyroidism. Treatment mainly involves correction of general condition.

STATION 5: MEDICAL DISORDERS WITH PREGNANCY

Thrombocytopenia with pregnancy

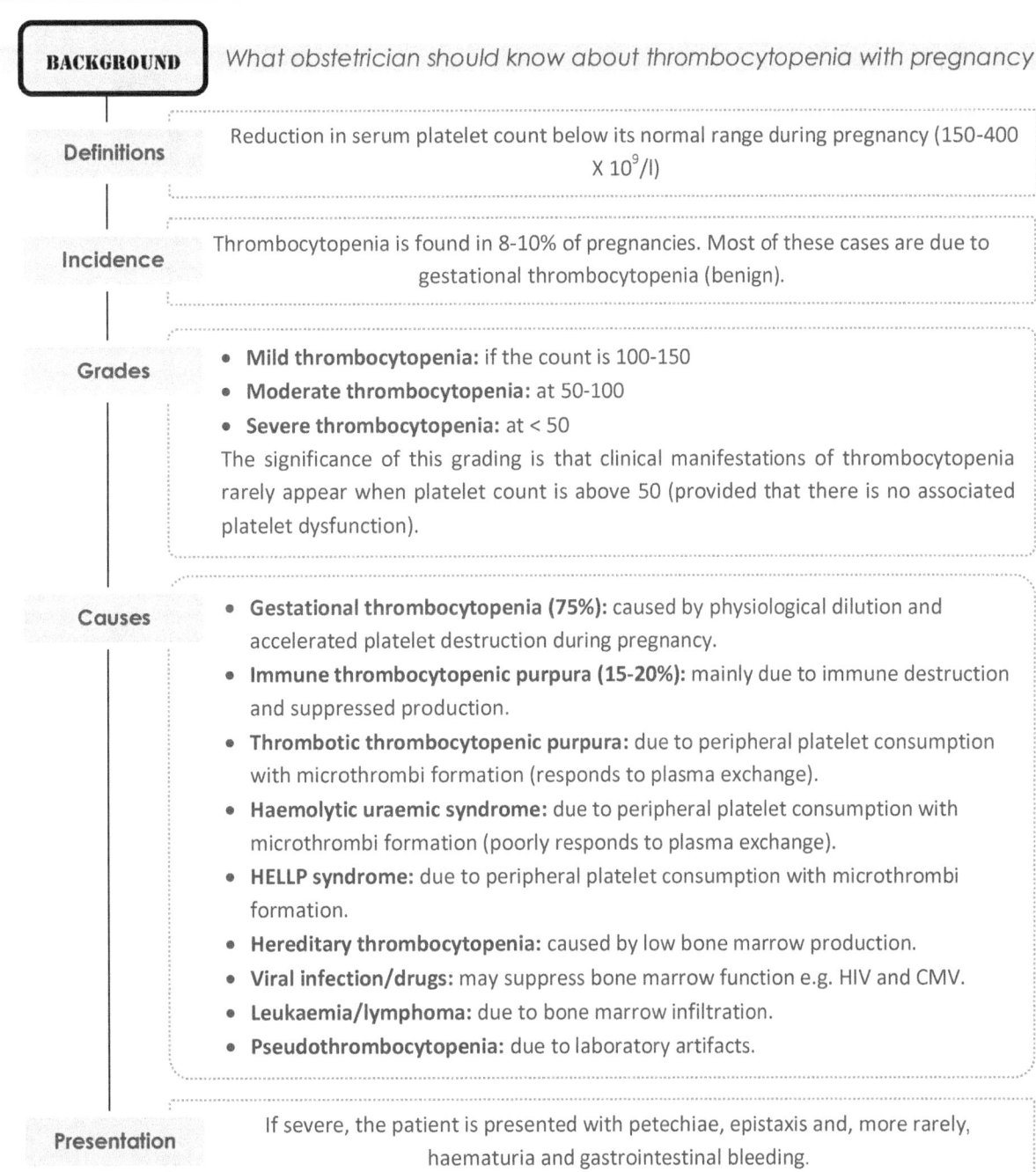

BACKGROUND — *What obstetrician should know about thrombocytopenia with pregnancy*

Definitions
Reduction in serum platelet count below its normal range during pregnancy (150-400 $\times 10^9$/l)

Incidence
Thrombocytopenia is found in 8-10% of pregnancies. Most of these cases are due to gestational thrombocytopenia (benign).

Grades
- **Mild thrombocytopenia:** if the count is 100-150
- **Moderate thrombocytopenia:** at 50-100
- **Severe thrombocytopenia:** at < 50

The significance of this grading is that clinical manifestations of thrombocytopenia rarely appear when platelet count is above 50 (provided that there is no associated platelet dysfunction).

Causes
- **Gestational thrombocytopenia (75%):** caused by physiological dilution and accelerated platelet destruction during pregnancy.
- **Immune thrombocytopenic purpura (15-20%):** mainly due to immune destruction and suppressed production.
- **Thrombotic thrombocytopenic purpura:** due to peripheral platelet consumption with microthrombi formation (responds to plasma exchange).
- **Haemolytic uraemic syndrome:** due to peripheral platelet consumption with microthrombi formation (poorly responds to plasma exchange).
- **HELLP syndrome:** due to peripheral platelet consumption with microthrombi formation.
- **Hereditary thrombocytopenia:** caused by low bone marrow production.
- **Viral infection/drugs:** may suppress bone marrow function e.g. HIV and CMV.
- **Leukaemia/lymphoma:** due to bone marrow infiltration.
- **Pseudothrombocytopenia:** due to laboratory artifacts.

Presentation
If severe, the patient is presented with petechiae, epistaxis and, more rarely, haematuria and gastrointestinal bleeding.

APPROACH *How obstetricians should deal with thrombocytopenia in pregnancy*

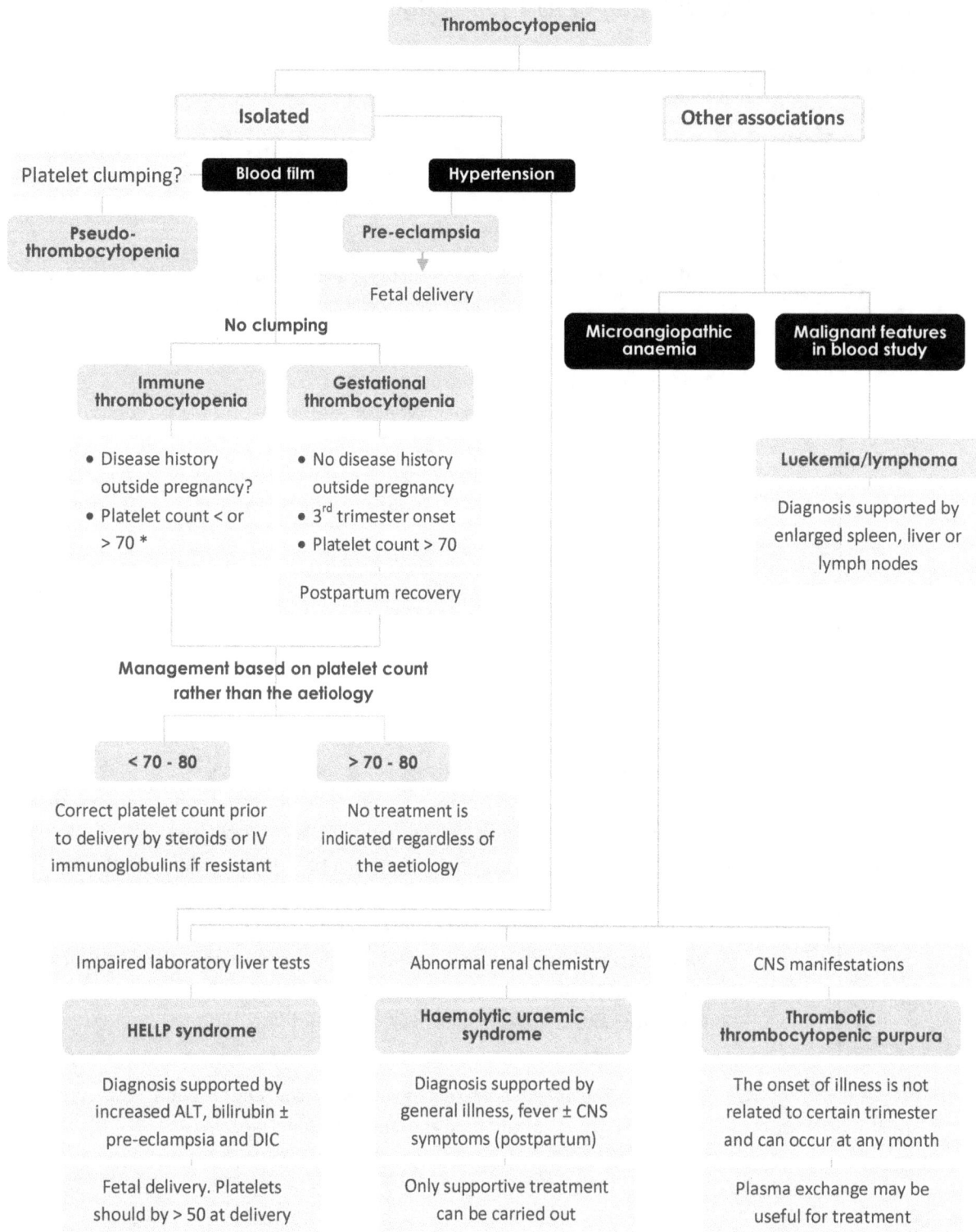

Thrombocytopenia

Isolated

Other associations

Platelet clumping? **Blood film** **Hypertension**

Pseudo-thrombocytopenia

Pre-eclampsia

Fetal delivery

No clumping

Microangiopathic anaemia **Malignant features in blood study**

Immune thrombocytopenia **Gestational thrombocytopenia**

Luekemia/lymphoma

- Disease history outside pregnancy?
- Platelet count < or > 70 *

- No disease history outside pregnancy
- 3rd trimester onset
- Platelet count > 70

Postpartum recovery

Diagnosis supported by enlarged spleen, liver or lymph nodes

Management based on platelet count rather than the aetiology

< 70 - 80 > 70 - 80

Correct platelet count prior to delivery by steroids or IV immunoglobulins if resistant

No treatment is indicated regardless of the aetiology

Impaired laboratory liver tests Abnormal renal chemistry CNS manifestations

HELLP syndrome **Haemolytic uraemic syndrome** **Thrombotic thrombocytopenic purpura**

Diagnosis supported by increased ALT, bilirubin ± pre-eclampsia and DIC

Fetal delivery. Platelets should by > 50 at delivery

Diagnosis supported by general illness, fever ± CNS symptoms (postpartum)

Only supportive treatment can be carried out

The onset of illness is not related to certain trimester and can occur at any month

Plasma exchange may be useful for treatment

* Immune thrombocytopenia is not diagnosed by detection of antibodies (poor sensitivity or specificity). Bone marrow aspiration is rarely needed (for unresponsive cases).

Fact Box: Criteria of gestational thrombocytopenia (diagnosis by exclusion)

- **During pregnancy:**
  - Mild thrombocytopenia (platelet count > 70 X 10^9/l)
  - No maternal symptoms (bleeding)
  - No past history of thrombocytopenia (before pregnancy)
  - Diagnosed in the third trimester
- **After delivery:**
  - No fetal thrombocytopenia
  - Spontaneous resolution after delivery
  - Recurrence in subsequent pregnancies is possible

A platelet count should be performed 6 weeks postnatally and the results should be reported.

Fact Box: Management of gestational thrombocytopenia

- **If platelet count is > 80:**
  No specific management is required. Delivery is managed as usual.
- **If platelet count 50-70:**
  - *Maternal concerns:*
    - Steroids should be tried.
    - Anaesthetic consultation for analgesic options during labour is essential. Epidural anaesthesia may not be recommended by most.
    - Cesarean section is done only on clear indications.
  - *Fetal/neonatal concerns:*
    - Fetal scalp electrodes or sampling are avoided.
    - High- or mid-cavity operative delivery are avoided.
    - Cord sampling is done to exclude neonatal thrombocytopenia.
    - Neonatal samples to recheck are taken at day 1 and 4.

Immune thrombocytopenic purpura

The incidence is 0.1–1/1000 pregnancies, 3% of cases of thrombocytopenia in pregnancy.

Pre-pregnancy counseling

Two thirds of cases are diagnosed prior to pregnancy.

- **Disease course:** it may relapse or worsen during pregnancy.
- **Safety:** If treatment is indicated, it carries maternal and fetal risks. One-third of women will require treatment, most commonly around the time of delivery.
- **Labour challenges:** There is an increased but small risk of haemorrhage at delivery even with low platelet count. Epidural anaesthesia may be contraindicated. Maternal deaths or serious complications are rare.
- **Neonatal risk:** unpredictable. However, higher risk is associated with thrombocytopenia in a sibling or the mother has undergone splenectomy. The risk of intracranial haemorrhage for the fetus/neonate is very low.

Antenatal care

Combined obstetric/hematology setting

- **Exclusion:** exclude other causes of thrombocytopenia as detailed before. Both gestational and immune thrombocytopenia are difficult to differentiate but both will be managed in the same way.
- **Follow up platelet count:** most cases will not require treatment during antenatal care.

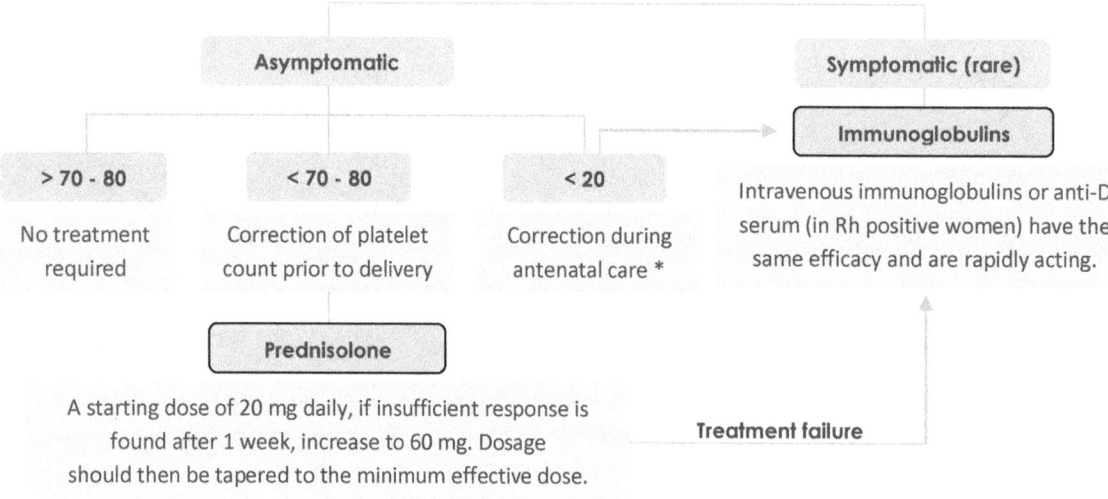

Asymptomatic

| > 70 - 80 | < 70 - 80 | < 20 |

No treatment required

Correction of platelet count prior to delivery

Correction during antenatal care *

Prednisolone

A starting dose of 20 mg daily, if insufficient response is found after 1 week, increase to 60 mg. Dosage should then be tapered to the minimum effective dose.

Symptomatic (rare)

Immunoglobulins

Intravenous immunoglobulins or anti-D serum (in Rh positive women) have the same efficacy and are rapidly acting.

Treatment failure

* During pregnancy, you do not have to keep platelet count but just above 20×10^9/l except if invasive procedures are indicated

Labour management

Close consultation with a haematologist experienced in obstetrics during labour

Check platelet count

Safe count for vaginal delivery should be > 40×10^9 and > 50×10^9 for operative/instrumental delivery

Delivery mode decision

Vaginal delivery is the safest route. Cesarean section should be selected on clear indications (CS does not decrease the risk intracranial haemorrhage in newborns)

Anaesthesia

Safe count for epidural anaesthesia > 80
Alternative analgesia for delivery needs anaesthetic consultation better in later pregnancy

Labour management

Fetal scalp electrodes or sampling and high- or mid-cavity operative delivery should be avoided to minimize the risk of intracranial haemorrhage of the newborn

Newborn management

The neonatal team should be alerted to the possibility of neonatal thrombocytopenia *

Cord blood sampling

Low platelets?

Confirm by Capillary sample

5% have count < 20 & 10% have count from 20-50

Do not give IM vitamin K before the count

Normal

No further management required

Mild thrombocytopenia

Repeat samples at day 1 and 4

Severe thrombocytopenia

IV immunoglobulin given + platelets if there is life-threatening haemorrhage

Consider cranial Doppler

* Fetal/neonatal thrombocytopenia is a possible risk due to trans-placental passage of maternal IgG to the fetus. This can cause intracranial haemorrhage which is rare but serious (< 1%). Neonatal thrombocytopenia (14-37%) cannot be predicted by maternal thrombocytopenia and is not affected by steroids or intravenous immunoglobulin and should not be diagnosed by fetal scalp samples or percutaneous umbilical blood sampling (risk of bleeding and death, 2%). Possible predictors may include affected siblings, maternal count < 50 or history of splenectomy.

Pre-eclampsia

15% of pre-eclampsia patients have thrombocytopenic count. 5% have severe thrombocytopenia

- **Mild or moderate pre-eclampsia:** conservative management may be appropriate.
- **Severe thrombocytopenia:** delivery is indicated.
- **Associated disseminated intravascular coagulation (with severe cases):** immediate management with fresh frozen plasma, cryoprecipitate and platelet transfusions.

The condition resolves quickly after delivery,

HELLP syndrome

10% of severe pre-eclampsia patients show HELLP syndrome. It may be complicated with DIC

- **Termination of pregnancy:** by fetal delivery is the mainstay of treatment for the mother. Neonatal outcome depends on the gestation age at delivery (10–20% die for very early delivery) and fetal growth restriction that is common. The platelet count should be maintained at >50.
  - Delivery may be indicated at any time from 20 weeks of gestation according to maternal condition or fetal condition (e.g. severe fetal growth restriction).
  - Conservative management for very early HELLP is controversial. Maternal risk versus fetal benefit should be weighed carefully.
- **Steroids:** should be given to enhance fetal lung maturity.
- **If DIC develops:** supportive care with fresh frozen plasma with or without cryoprecipitate.

The condition improves immediately after delivery. However, it may worsen during the first 24–48 hours postpartum.

Thrombotic thrombocytopenic purpura

Severe deficiency of von Willebrand's factor-cleaving protein (ADAMTS 13) occurs in 1:25 000 pregnancies (at any time but 55% of cases occur in the second trimester)

- **Plasma exchange:** should be commenced urgently even if the diagnosis is difficult to confirm.
  This treatment removes antibodies, 1–1.5 l fresh frozen plasma containing the defective enzyme is given daily until platelet count is corrected and the lactate dehydrogenase is reduced.
- **High doses of steroids:** may be indicated.
- **Rituximab (monoclonal antibody against CD20):** is useful when improvement is slow.
- **Fresh frozen plasma:** is used instead of plasma exchange in the rare congenital cases (no antibodies in this variety).
- **Platelet transfusions:** are contraindicated (precipitate or exacerbate CNS symptoms).

About 25% of women suffer recurrent episodes. Predictors of relapse include previous clinical presentation and low ADAMTS13 during remission.

Appendix   **Fetal and neonatal thrombocytopenia**

Causes of fetal/neonatal thrombocytopenia

- **Maternal ITP:** placental crossing of maternal IgG antibodies.
- **Fetal infections of the fetus:** may cause thrombocytopenia.
- **Fetal and neonatal alloimmune thrombocytopenia (FNAIT):**
    - *Definition:* this is a serious condition in which is there are antigens on fetal platelets that are not present on the maternal platelets. These antigens stimulate maternal antibody formation that causes platelet destruction.
    - *Presentation:* this may be complicated by intracranial haemorrhage (26% - 80% occur before birth).
    - *Management:*
        - Early diagnosis and treatment using matched platelets.
        - High doses of intravenous immunoglobulin ± prednisolone (0.5 g/kg).
        - Serial fetal platelet transfusions.
        - Counseling the parents for possible recurrence.

STATION 5: MEDICAL DISORDERS WITH PREGNANCY

Sickle Cell Disease in Pregnancy

BACKGROUND   *What obstetrician should know about Sickle Cell Disease in Pregnancy*

Definitions

Sickle cell disease is an inherited autosomal recessive disorders caused by single gene mutation involving haemoglobin structure.

This mutation causes the formation of abnormal haemoglobin in low-oxygen conditions, red cells become rigid and fragile with subsequent haemolytic anaemia, and vaso-occlusion in the small blood vessels.

Types

Homozygous   This is called sickle cell anaemia (HbSS). This gives the typical picture of the disease

Heterozygous   Combination with haemoglobin C (HbSC)   Similar clinical
Combination with beta thalassaemia (HbSB)   picture with
Combination with haemoglobin D, E or O-Arab   varying severity

Combination with normal haemoglobin (A),   Asymptomatic
This is called sickle trait (HbAS)   except for
increased risk of
UT infections and
microscopic
haematuria

Incidence

- The disease is most common in African descent, in the Caribbean, Middle East, parts of India and the Mediterranean, and South and Central America.
- It is the most common inherited condition worldwide (300 000 children per year - two-thirds are in Africa).
- In the UK, 300 children with SCD are born per year, 100–200 women with SCD get pregnant per year in the UK.

Complications

- Haemolytic anaemia.
- Vaso-occlusion in the small blood vessels and acute painful crises.
- Stroke, pulmonary hypertension, renal dysfunction, retinal disease and leg ulcers.
- Cholelithiasis.
- Avascular necrosis (the femoral head is commonly affected).

APPROACH   *How obstetricians should deal with Sickle Cell Disease in Pregnancy*

I. Pre-conception care

Document woman's intentions regarding contraception or conception in each contact with her sickle cell team

Counseling

Sickle specialist

The specialist is concerned about counseling the woman for (see later):
- How pregnancy affects sickle cell disease
- How to improve fetal and maternal outcomes (optimal management)
- How to screen for end organ damage

Advice and care

Primary care physician

The primary health physician should play a role in the following:
- Preconceptual screening (see later)
- Supply general pre-conception care
- Advise about vaccinations, medications and crisis avoidance

Willing to use contraception?

A primary health physician is involved on provision of contraceptive advice

Willing to conceive?

Counseling for possible maternal and fetal risks

Genetic screening

A primary health physician is involved in partner screening and genetic counseling. Advise testing the haemoglobinopathy status of the partner

Not available

Consider the fetus as high risk

Available

HbS or β thalassaemia O-Arab, HbC or D-Punjab	DB thalassaemia Lepore, HbE or HPFH *
Refer for counselling - offer prenatal diagnosis	Counselling – possible further investigations

Methods and risks of prenatal diagnosis and termination of pregnancy are discussed with the couple

Medications

Antibiotics/vaccines are administered and monitored in primary care but reviewed by haematologist/obstetrician during pregnancy

Prophylaxis

Daily penicillin prophylaxis – Erythromycin in case of allergy (SCD is hyposplenic state)

H. influenza type b, the conjugated meningococcal C vaccine (single dose), pneumococcal vaccine (every 5 years). Hepatitis B vaccine is given. Influenza and swine flu vaccine (annually)

Folic acid

1 mg/day outside pregnancy, 5 mg preconception & during pregnancy

Modifications

Hydroxyurea is stopped 3 months prior to conception**. ACEIs are also stopped.

---

* Hereditary persistence of fetal hemoglobin (HPFH)

** If pregnancy occurs while on treatment, do not terminate but offer level 3 ultrasound for fetal anomalies.

Counseling women with SCD who plan to conceive (RCOG)

- Inform women about factors that participate sickle cell crises e.g. dehydration, cold, hypoxia, overexertion and stress. This includes nausea and vomiting in pregnancy due to dehydration.
- Inform about the risk of worsening anaemia, the increased risk of crises and acute chest syndrome (ACS) and the risk of increased infection (urinary tract infection) during pregnancy.
- Inform about the increased risk of fetal growth restriction, fetal distress, induction of labour and caesarean section. Risk of SCD in the offspring should be discussed.

Screening women with SCD for disease complications	
Screening for pulmonary hypertension	• Screening is carried out with echocardiography. • The risk is higher with SCD. Screening is performed if no screening has been done in the last year. • Tricuspid regurgitant jet velocity > 2.5 m/second is associated with a high risk of pulmonary hypertension.
Screening for hypertension, renal and hepatic complications	• Blood pressure and urinalysis is performed to screen for hypertension and/or proteinuria. • Renal and liver function tests are performed annually for sickle nephropathy and/or hepatic complications.
Retinal screening	Preconception retinal screening is recommended because proliferative retinopathy is common in patients with SCD, especially patients with HbSC.
Screening for iron loading (women with repeated transfusions)	• High ferritin level and T2 cardiac magnetic resonance imaging helps to assess iron loading. • If a woman is heavily loaded with iron, aggressive iron chelation before conception is recommended.
Screening for red cell antibodies	Red cell antibodies are screened because they are associated with an increased risk of haemolytic disease of the newborn.

Consider multidisciplinary team including high-risk pregnancy experienced obstetrician, midwife, and a haematologist

II. Antenatal care

First appointment		
Primary care or hospital appointment		

Counseling and providing information
- Counsel the couple and offer partner testing if this has not been achieved preconceptually.

Evaluating current clinical status
- Take a clinical history to assess the complications of SCD.
- Document baseline oxygen saturations and blood pressure.
- Offer retinal, renal and cardiac assessments (if not performed in the last year).
- Send midstream urine for culture.

Reviewing current treatment
- Stop taking hydroxycarbamide, ACE inhibitors or ARBs.
- Advise taking 5 mg folic acid.
- Advise taking antibiotic prophylaxis.
- Discuss vaccinations.

7-9 weeks

Perform an ultrasound to confirm viability (risk of miscarriage) - assess gestational age

10 weeks (Booking appointment)

High-risk pregnancy experienced mid-wife

Counseling and providing information
- Counsel the woman about the effect of pregnancy on SCD and the potential maternal and fetal risks.
- Give clear information and advice including the crisis participating e.g. extreme temperatures, dehydration and overexertion and the risk of persistent vomiting.

Evaluating current clinical status
- Assess renal function test, urine protein/creatinine ratio, liver function test and ferritin.
- Assess extended red cell phenotype.

Reviewing test results & treatment
- Review partner genetic results. Discuss further steps according to the results including the risks and benefits of prenatal diagnosis if indicated.
- Consider low dose aspirin from the 12th week of gestation. Iron is given only if indicated (iron deficiency).

16 weeks
Mid-wife and multidisciplinary team

Routine antenatal care - Repeat midstream urine culture - Multidisciplinary check (consultant obstetrician and haematologist)

20 weeks
Mid-wife and multidisciplinary team

Detailed fetal ultrasound scanning - Repeat midstream urine culture – repeat fetal blood count

24 weeks
Multidisciplinary team

Ultrasound monitoring and follow up of fetal growth and amniotic fluid - Repeat midstream urine culture

26 weeks
Mid-wife

Routine antenatal care visit with routine check including measurement of blood pressure and assessment of proteinuria

28 weeks **Multidisciplinary team**	Ultrasound monitoring and follow up of fetal growth and amniotic fluid - Repeat midstream urine culture – Repeat fetal blood count, group and antibody screen
30 weeks **Mid-wife – ANC classes**	Routine antenatal care visit with routine check including measurement of blood pressure and assessment of proteinuria
32 weeks **Multidisciplinary team**	Routine antenatal check visit - Ultrasound monitoring and follow up of fetal growth and amniotic fluid - Repeat midstream urine culture – Repeat fetal blood count
34 weeks **Mid-wife**	Routine antenatal care visit with routine check including measurement of blood pressure and assessment of proteinuria

36 weeks
Multidisciplinary team

Evaluating current clinical status	• Routine antenatal check visit • Ultrasound monitoring and follow up of fetal growth and amniotic fluid
Counseling and providing information	• Discuss timing, mode and management of the birth • Discuss analgesia and anaesthesia; arrange anaesthetic assessment • Offer information about baby care after birth

38 weeks **Mid-wife - obstetrician**	Routine ANC check - Discuss induction of labour or caesarean section between 38 and 40 weeks of gestation
39 weeks **Mid-wife**	Offer routine ANC check – Advise the woman and arrange to deliver by 40 weeks of gestation
40 weeks Obstetrician	Offer routine ANC check – Offer fetal monitoring if the woman declines delivery by 40 weeks of gestation

Management of complications

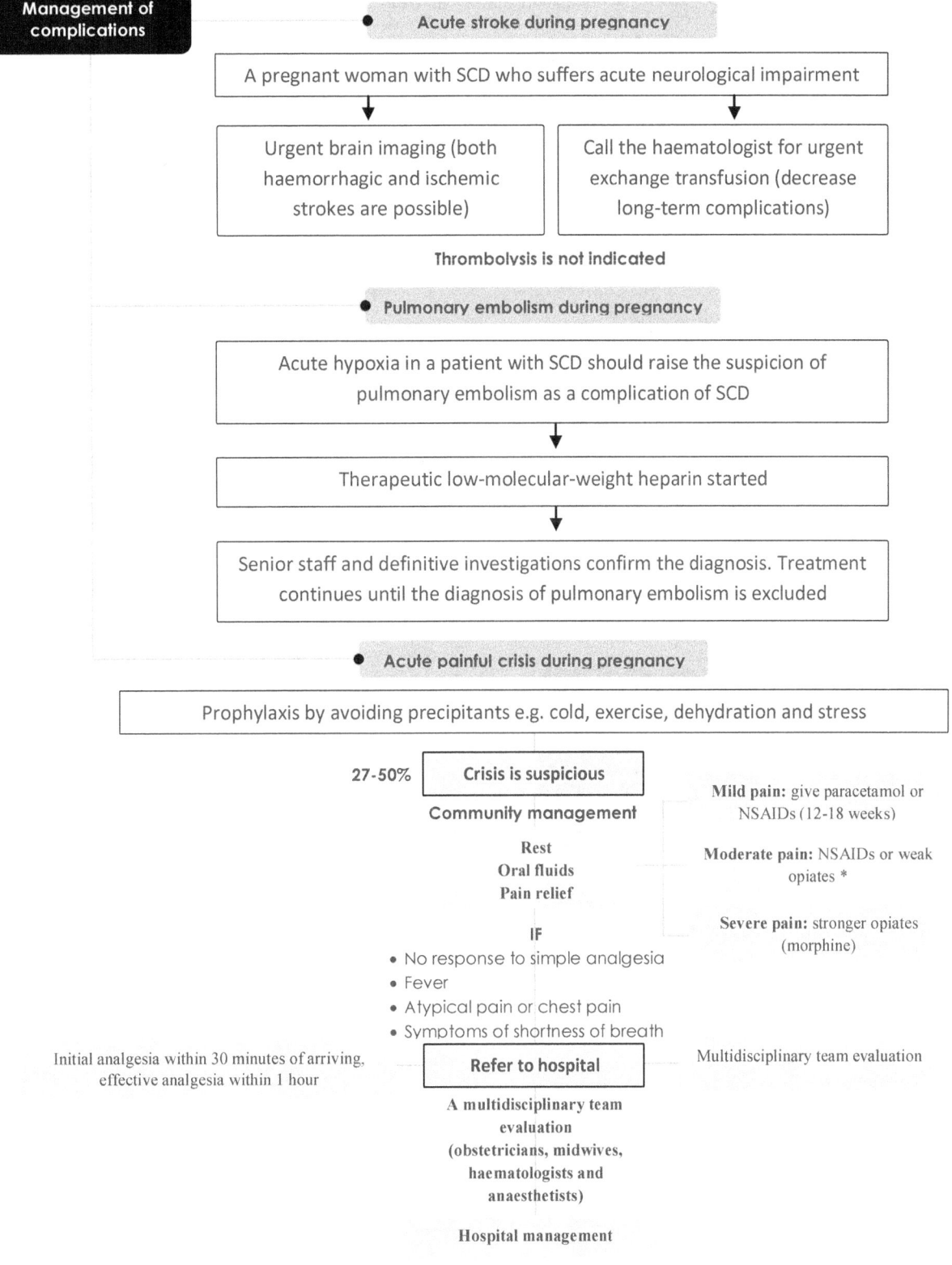

● **Acute stroke during pregnancy**

A pregnant woman with SCD who suffers acute neurological impairment

Urgent brain imaging (both haemorrhagic and ischemic strokes are possible)

Call the haematologist for urgent exchange transfusion (decrease long-term complications)

Thrombolysis is not indicated

● **Pulmonary embolism during pregnancy**

Acute hypoxia in a patient with SCD should raise the suspicion of pulmonary embolism as a complication of SCD

Therapeutic low-molecular-weight heparin started

Senior staff and definitive investigations confirm the diagnosis. Treatment continues until the diagnosis of pulmonary embolism is excluded

● **Acute painful crisis during pregnancy**

Prophylaxis by avoiding precipitants e.g. cold, exercise, dehydration and stress

27-50% **Crisis is suspicious**

Community management

Rest
Oral fluids
Pain relief

IF
- No response to simple analgesia
- Fever
- Atypical pain or chest pain
- Symptoms of shortness of breath

Initial analgesia within 30 minutes of arriving, effective analgesia within 1 hour

Refer to hospital

A multidisciplinary team evaluation (obstetricians, midwives, haematologists and anaesthetists)

Hospital management

Mild pain: give paracetamol or NSAIDs (12-18 weeks)

Moderate pain: NSAIDs or weak opiates *

Severe pain: stronger opiates (morphine)

Multidisciplinary team evaluation

* Weak opioids include co-dydramol, co-codamol or dihydrocodeine. Pethidine should be avoided because of the risk of toxicity and seizures in SCD.

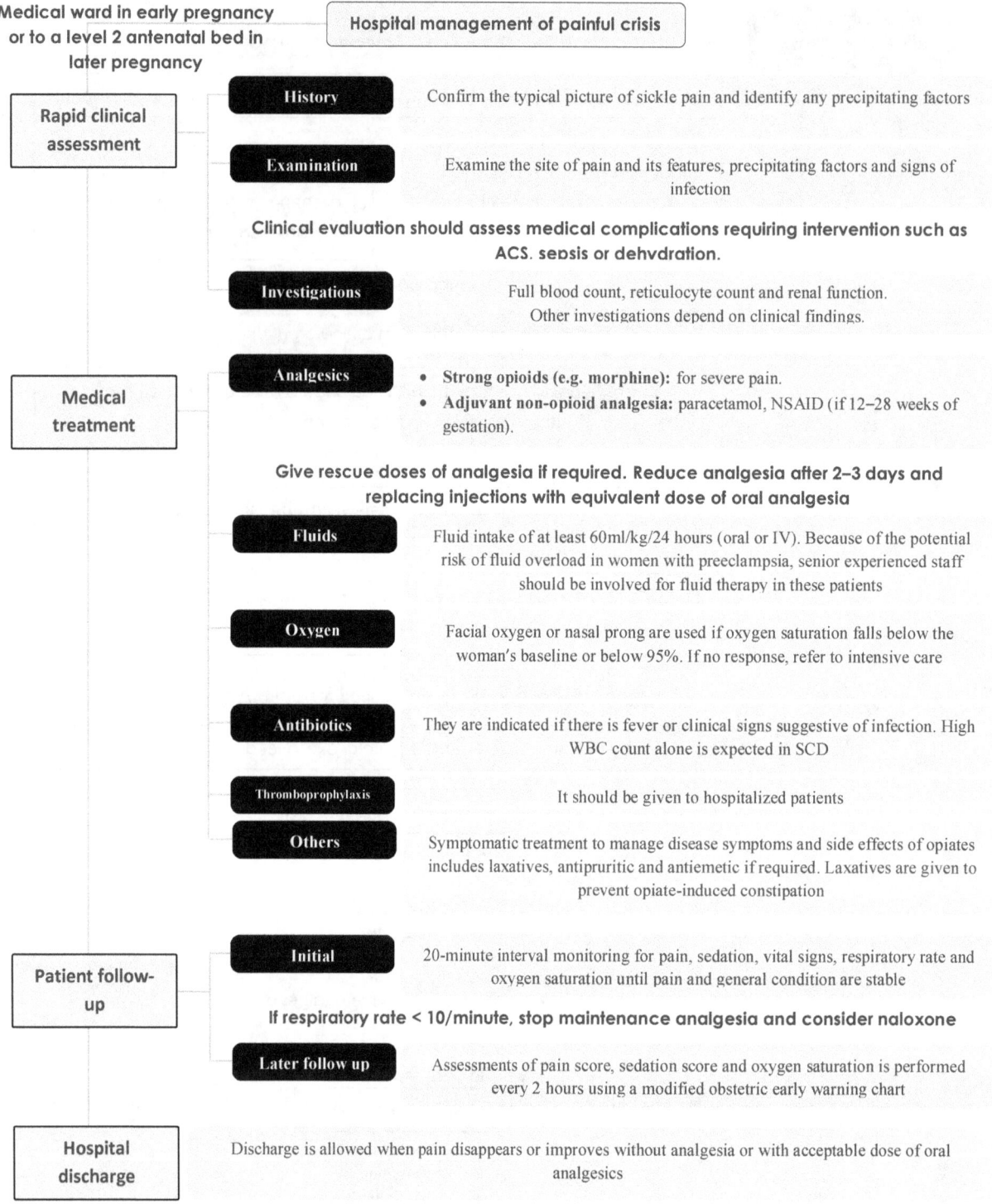

Medical ward in early pregnancy or to a level 2 antenatal bed in later pregnancy

Hospital management of painful crisis

Rapid clinical assessment

History — Confirm the typical picture of sickle pain and identify any precipitating factors

Examination — Examine the site of pain and its features, precipitating factors and signs of infection

Clinical evaluation should assess medical complications requiring intervention such as ACS, sepsis or dehydration.

Investigations — Full blood count, reticulocyte count and renal function. Other investigations depend on clinical findings.

Medical treatment

Analgesics —
- **Strong opioids (e.g. morphine):** for severe pain.
- **Adjuvant non-opioid analgesia:** paracetamol, NSAID (if 12–28 weeks of gestation).

Give rescue doses of analgesia if required. Reduce analgesia after 2–3 days and replacing injections with equivalent dose of oral analgesia

Fluids — Fluid intake of at least 60ml/kg/24 hours (oral or IV). Because of the potential risk of fluid overload in women with preeclampsia, senior experienced staff should be involved for fluid therapy in these patients

Oxygen — Facial oxygen or nasal prong are used if oxygen saturation falls below the woman's baseline or below 95%. If no response, refer to intensive care

Antibiotics — They are indicated if there is fever or clinical signs suggestive of infection. High WBC count alone is expected in SCD

Thromboprophylaxis — It should be given to hospitalized patients

Others — Symptomatic treatment to manage disease symptoms and side effects of opiates includes laxatives, antipruritic and antiemetic if required. Laxatives are given to prevent opiate-induced constipation

Patient follow-up

Initial — 20-minute interval monitoring for pain, sedation, vital signs, respiratory rate and oxygen saturation until pain and general condition are stable

If respiratory rate < 10/minute, stop maintenance analgesia and consider naloxone

Later follow up — Assessments of pain score, sedation score and oxygen saturation is performed every 2 hours using a modified obstetric early warning chart

Hospital discharge — Discharge is allowed when pain disappears or improves without analgesia or with acceptable dose of oral analgesics

---

* Morphine or diamorphine can be given by the oral, subcutaneous, intramuscular or intravenous route. Parenteral opiates can be given by intermittent bolus or patient-controlled systems. This depends on woman's preference. Opiates are not associated with teratogenicity or congenital malformation. They may cause transient suppression of fetal movement and a reduced baseline fetal heart variability. Observe the neonate for signs of opiate withdrawal if the mother receives prolonged course of opiates in late pregnancy.

Management of complications (cont)

7-20%

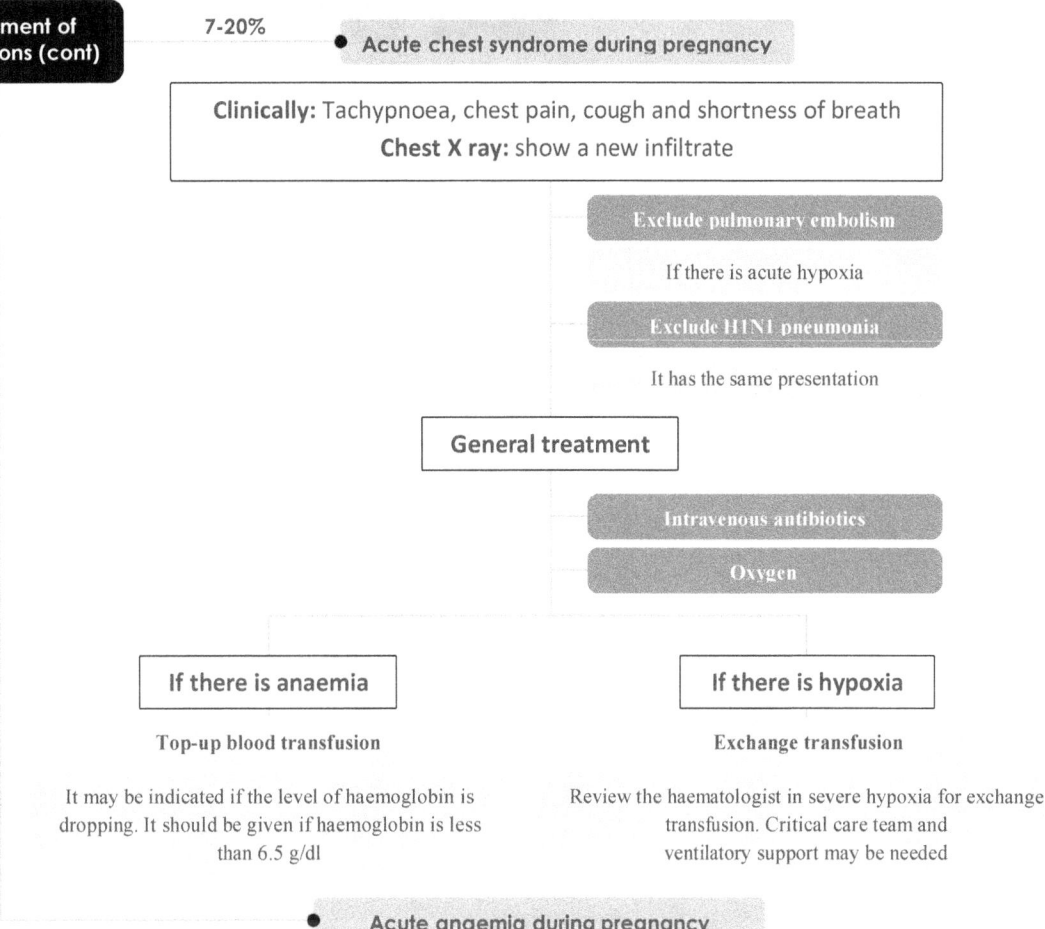

● **Acute chest syndrome during pregnancy**

Clinically: Tachypnoea, chest pain, cough and shortness of breath
Chest X ray: show a new infiltrate

Exclude pulmonary embolism

If there is acute hypoxia

Exclude H1N1 pneumonia

It has the same presentation

General treatment

Intravenous antibiotics

Oxygen

If there is anaemia

Top-up blood transfusion

It may be indicated if the level of haemoglobin is dropping. It should be given if haemoglobin is less than 6.5 g/dl

If there is hypoxia

Exchange transfusion

Review the haematologist in severe hypoxia for exchange transfusion. Critical care team and ventilatory support may be needed

● **Acute anaemia during pregnancy**

- Blood transfusion
- Woman isolation
- Consider reticulocyte count:
    - <u>Low count</u>: this may indicate aplastic crisis caused by erythrovirus (a cause of hydrops fetalis) - Refer to a fetal medicine specialist.
    - <u>High count</u>: indicates hemolytic crisis.

III. Intrapartum care

Pre-labour assessment and considerations

- Advise and arrange for the place of birth. Hospitals that can manage high-risk pregnancies and complications of SCD (e.g. abruption, pre-eclampsia, peripartum cardiomyopathy and acute sickle cell crisis) are recommended.
- Discuss suitable positioning during fetal delivery in women who had hip replacements due to avascular necrosis
- Anaesthetic assessment is performed in the third trimester.

Smooth maternal course and normal fetal growth?

Pregnancy is 38+0 weeks or more

Elective birth

- *Blood preparation:*
  - Cross-matched blood if atypical antibodies are present (saves time).
  - A 'group and save' if there are no atypical antibodies.
- *Multidisciplinary team:*
  A senior midwife, senior obstetrician, anaesthetist and haematologist are notified once labour is confirmed.

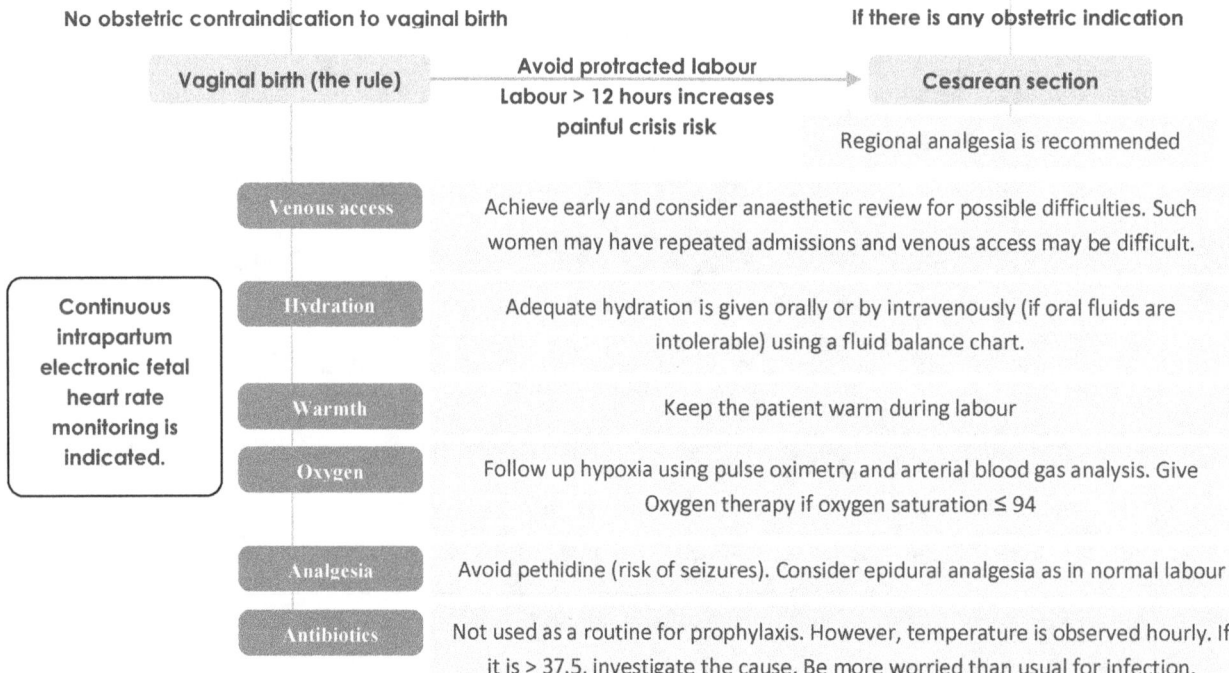

No obstetric contraindication to vaginal birth   **If there is any obstetric indication**

Vaginal birth (the rule) → **Avoid protracted labour** / Labour > 12 hours increases painful crisis risk → **Cesarean section**

Regional analgesia is recommended

Continuous intrapartum electronic fetal heart rate monitoring is indicated.

Venous access	Achieve early and consider anaesthetic review for possible difficulties. Such women may have repeated admissions and venous access may be difficult.
Hydration	Adequate hydration is given orally or by intravenously (if oral fluids are intolerable) using a fluid balance chart.
Warmth	Keep the patient warm during labour
Oxygen	Follow up hypoxia using pulse oximetry and arterial blood gas analysis. Give Oxygen therapy if oxygen saturation ≤ 94
Analgesia	Avoid pethidine (risk of seizures). Consider epidural analgesia as in normal labour
Antibiotics	Not used as a routine for prophylaxis. However, temperature is observed hourly. If it is > 37.5, investigate the cause. Be more worried than usual for infection.

IV. Postpartum care

The probability of complications of SCD including acute crisis continues during puerperium. The risk of sickle cell crisis is 25% and is more after general anaesthesia. Accordingly, the same level of care and caution that is considered during pregnancy should continue during puerperium

Maternal care

Oxygen/hydration

Give adequate hydration (according to fluid balance) and oxygen (oxygen saturation < 94%) until discharge.

Mobilization

Encourage early mobilization of the patient

Breast-feeding

Allow and encourage breast-feeding (as normal puerperium)

Thromboprophylaxis

Low-molecular-weight heparin is given during hospitalization and 7 days post-discharge (after vaginal delivery) or 6 weeks (after caesarean section).

Antithrombotic stockings are recommended during puerperium.

NSAIDS

They are given routinely during puerperium and they are not contraindicated during breast-feeding.

Newborn care

Consider early newborn testing using capillary sample if the father is a carrier or a patient

Contraception

- Progestogen-containing contraceptives (bills, injectables and intrauterine system) are the first line.
- Estrogen-containing contraceptives are second-line agents (theoretical risk of venous thromboembolism in these women).
- Copper IUD devices are also second line agents

Appendix   **Indications of transfusion during pregnancy**

Blood transfusion during pregnancy

Routine prophylactic transfusion is not recommended.

Women with previous medical, fetal or obstetric complications	Women on transfusion regimen to prevent complications	Women with multiple pregnancies	Women with acute anaemia	Women with acute chest pain or acute stroke
Exchange or top-up transfusion (multi-disciplinary decision)	Transfusion should be continued during pregnancy	Prophylactic transfusion (these women are at higher risk of complications)	Top-up transfusion	Exchange transfusion

- Blood used for transfusion should be cytomegalovirus negative.
- Blood should be matched for full rhesus typing (C, D and E) and Kell typing (an extended phenotype). Alloimmunisation is common in SCD.

STATION 5: MEDICAL DISORDERS WITH PREGNANCY

Cardiac Diseases in Pregnancy

> **BACKGROUND**   *What obstetrician should know about cardiac diseases in Pregnancy*

Varieties

Myocardial infarction, ischaemic heart disease

- **Risks of myocardial infarction during pregnancy:**

  ❶ Pregnancy itself:

  - Pregnancy itself increases the risk of acute myocardial infarction by 3 to 4-fold.
  - The risk being 30 times higher for women > 40 years compared with women < 20 years.

  ❷ Other risk factors (general risk factors): Chronic hypertension, pre-eclampsia, diabetes, smoking, obesity and hyperlipidaemia.

- **Prognosis:** The risk of death in women with myocardial infarction is Up to 1/13.

Peripartum cardiomyopathy

There is no identifiable cause or risk factors for this serious condition. Accordingly, it should be suspected in every pregnant woman complaining of cardiac symptoms in late pregnancy or early in the puerperium. However, it may occur up to 6 months after delivery.

Rheumatic heart disease

Women who live in developing countries (or originated in these countries) may never have undergone medical screening. Those who have rheumatic heart disease may be unaware of their problem before pregnancy. Accordingly, a careful cardiovascular assessment for these women including auscultation of the heart is highly important.

Aortic dissection

Blood pressure monitoring and proper control using antihypertensive therapy during pregnancy is the most important approach in these cases because systolic hypertension is the most important risk implicated in deaths from aortic dissection.

Congenital heart disease

The prevalence of congenital heart disease in pregnancy is about 0.8%. However, death from this group of diseases is uncommon.

Risk of death

Myocardial infarction	One third of maternal deaths due to heart diseases
Peripartum cardiomyopathy	One third of maternal deaths due to heart diseases
Others	Rheumatic heart disease, congenital heart disease and pulmonary hypertension contribute by 5-10% each.

APPROACH   *How obstetricians should deal with cardiac Diseases in Pregnancy*

I. Pre-conception care

A girl with heart disease approximating teenage
(typically 12 - 15 years)

Joint cardiac, obstetric,
gynaecological team assessment
(expertise in cardiac diseases with
pregnancy)

Older women with
new diagnosis

Advise specialist care from a high-
risk pregnancy with heart disease
team in future pregnancy.

Give an outline of the issues relating
to pregnancy with congenital heart
disease at the first visit

Estimate the risk accurately and
review it every five years (or
according to general condition).

The girl does not
consider conception?

The girl considers
conception?

Avoiding unwanted pregnancy is the main concern.
Discuss contraceptive options

Give more detailed review about cardiac disease in
pregnancy supported with a simple information
leaflet. The review includes the increased risk of
mortality, congenital heart disease in the offspring
and the need for increased medical surveillance
during pregnancy.

Natural methods	Safe method - Unreliable when pregnancy should be avoided.
Barrier methods	Few side effects - High failure rate.
IUCD and mirena	Effective, less bleeding & infection with mirena, Risk of syncope at insertion
Combined pills	Effective, risk of thrombosis particularly with thrombogenic heart diseases
Mini pills	No thrombosis, Desogestrel pills are more effective than traditional pills
Injectables	Effective, consider cardiac patients on warfarin
Implants	The most effective method, excellent safety profile, bosentan lessen effect
Sterilization	Male sterilization, minilaparotomy and hysteroscopic approaches are safer.

> **Contraceptive options for a cardiac patient - How to counsel and choose**

Natural methods

They are safe options. However, they are not suitable when unwanted pregnancy is serious because they are unreliable.

Barrier methods

They have few side effects and provide protection against sexually transmitted diseases. However, their failure rate is considerable.

IUCD and mirena

Copper IUCD and mirena are more reliable. Mirena is associated with less bleeding and infection. The main concern for cardiac patients is the rare but considerable risk of a fainting reaction during insertion (0.01%). Advise insertion in hospital and with a cardiac anaesthetic expertise on standby.

Combined pills

It is the most effective method. It also has many non-contraceptive advantages. However, there is 3 to 4-fold increase in the risk of thrombosis (1:5000 women a year, fatal in 25% of cases). Weighing benefits against risk, the risk of death from thrombosis is half the risk of death from getting pregnant. But combined pills are to be avoided in cardiac disease that are associated with clotting and thrombosis.

Mini pills

- Traditional low-dose pills: it is not associated with thrombosis. However, they have higher failure rate.
- Desogestrel containing pills (Cerazette®): they are more effective than the traditional pills. Irregular bleeding is a side effect of both.

Injectables

Depo-provera ® is a very effective and long-term option for contraception. A part from the irregular or heavy bleeding following discontinuation and needle phobia, cardiac patients on warfarin are usually not eligible.

Implants

Nexplanon is the most effective and one of the safest options for contraception. As with other methods containing progestins, bosentan (used by some cardiac patients) may reduce its effectiveness.

Sterilization

Male sterilization is safer and more effective. For female sterilization, mini-lapraotomy may be safer than laparoscopy (gas expansion) using regional anaesthesia (more suitable for cardiac patients). Hysteroscopic approach (Essure) is done under local anaesthetic or intravenous sedation and this is preferable in cardiac patients. However, it is not yet widely available.

II. Antenatal care

Identification of cardiac patients

Congenital heart disease → Most women with cardiac diseases know and follow up prior to pregnancy

Ischemic heart disease → The patient may have prior history of cardiac ischemia. However, any pregnant woman with chest pain should have ECG (electrocardiogram) interpreted by an expertise. Serum troponin may be useful particularly if the ECG is suspicious.

Aortic dissection → This complication should be suspected in women with Marphan syndrome. Furthermore, any woman with severe chest pain should be assessed using chest CT or MRI scan in addition to ECG.

Rheumatic heart disease → Many women may be discovered during pregnancy. Careful cardiac examination in the first antenatal care visit is essential for women originating from the developing countries. The most common affection is mitral stenosis (the highest risk). Clinical diagnosis may be difficult and careful echocardiography examination is indicated.

Peripartum cardiomyopathy → Any woman with increased shortness of breath, especially on lying flat or at night should be suspected. It should not be confused with pre-eclampsia (because hypertension is present in 25% of these patients). Assessment with electrocardiogram, chest X-ray and echocardiogram is essential.

Initial risk assessment

Any woman with cardiac disease or with murmurs on examination should be assessed for risk by a joint clinic (consultant obstetrician, cardiologist and anaesthetist with adequate experience) - Consider initial echo and ECG that will be kept as a reference

Significant risk	Low risk
Frequent antenatal care visits by an experienced OB consultant	Return to routine antenatal care

Frequency: Antenatal care visits are scheduled every 2-4 weeks until 20 weeks, then every 2 weeks until 24 weeks and then weekly according to her cardiac condition.

Content: Routine obstetric assessment + Cardiac assessment (later)

12 weeks	Nuchal translucency scan (may indicate recurrent cardiac disease)
20 weeks	Standard fetal anomaly scan
22 weeks	Fetal cardiac scan for women with congenital heart diseases (performed by fetal cardiologists versus fetal medicine specialist in normal pregnancy)
32-34 weeks	Multidisciplinary meeting to determine the plan of delivery
	Inform the woman about how to recognize the onset of labour
	Discuss the plan of labour (e.g. mode of delivery, bearing down)
	Discuss postpartum details including thromboprophylaxis

> **Cardiac assessment during antenatal care visits**

The main concern is to identify cardiac manifestations and to differentiate them from the normal tiredness of pregnancy

I. History

❶ Ask the woman how many flights of stairs she can afford without shortness of breath (woman's demeanour and way of answering may be more informative than the answer itself). Ask about palpitations

New York Heart association classification	Symptoms
I	No limitation of ordinary physical activity
II	Mild symptoms with ordinary activity
III	Marked symptoms, even with less-than-ordinary activity e.g. walking 20–100 m.
IV	Symptoms even while at rest.

❷ Sudden increase in shortness of breath or new palpitations should be carefully assessed with a cardiologist. The best initial assessment will be the ECG and an emergency echocardiography should be obtained.

II. Examination

Mini-exercise test

You may call a woman from the waiting room to your consulting room. See how quickly she can walk. Check her breath status her pulse rate and rhythm when she first sits down

Vital signs

- *Blood pressure:* is measured manually (woman is comfortable, not talking).
- *Pulse:* is measured for rate and rhythm (Increase pulse rate can be one of the first signs of cardiac decompensation). The pulse rate is best measured using by cardiac auscultation, when the pulse becomes fast, irregular or faint.

Heart auscultation

Check cardiac murmurs with each visit and compare them with previous records. Murmurs may normally increase by one grade (murmurs have 6 grades) due to increase blood flow through the heart. The following should be considered:

- A sudden increase in murmur intensity or development of new murmurs is suspicious for infective endocarditis.
- A diastolic murmur in a patient with Marphan syndrome indicates aortic regurge and carries the risk of aortic dissection or heart failure.

Lung auscultation

Auscultate the bases of the lungs posteriorly for possible crackles indicating pulmonary edema and hear failure. However, you should consider 2 points before jumping to a conclusion:

- Persistent crackles in a localised area may be a sequence of previous surgery, it should be reported early in pregnancy to avoid confusion.
- Crackles due to poor lung expansion may develop late in pregnancy by the pressure of the enlarging uterus. Avoid by asking the woman to take several deep breaths and cough several times. These crackles will disappear if not pathological.

Assess oxygen saturation at each trimester (or more frequent in indicated cases).
Advise the woman to have more rest than usual. However, motivate her to keep her fitness. Any abnormalities revealed with examination should be managed accordingly based on cardiac consultation

III. Intrapartum care

Counsel for labour

At 32-24 weeks of gestation, a multidisciplinary assessment is indicated. The following points about labour are discussed:

- Deciding who should be involved in labour observation.
- Deciding if a caesarean section is indicated.
- Deciding if bearing down is advisable in the second stage.
- Deciding how to guard against postpartum haemorrhage whether after vaginal delivery or Cesarean section.
- Deciding postpartum management plan (the appropriateness of thromboprophylaxis, the length of postpartum hospital stay, the timing of cardiac and obstetric review).

Arrange for a labour place

The decision about the place for antenatal and intrapartum care should be made by both the obstetrician and the cardiologist. A tertiary unit (specialized in the management of women with heart disease in pregnancy with high-dependency and intensive care units) is appropriate.

Labour approach at term

No obstetric contraindication to vaginal birth

Vaginal delivery

- Consider early slow incremental epidural anaesthesia to minimize the stress of pain
- Consider assisted vaginal delivery to cut short the stressful second stage

Protection against postpartum hemorrhage
Low-dose syntocinon infusion instead of routinely used oxytocic regimes

If there is any obstetric indication

Cesarean section

- Anaesthesia is provided by a senior staff

Protection against postpartum hemorrhage
Prophylactic uterine compression sutures can be considered instead of oxytocics due to their cardiovascular effect

IV. Postpartum care

- The length of recommended stay in hospital and the need for anticoagulation, the duration of observation in a high-dependency area and the timing of follow-up at the joint clinic should be determined prior to labour.
- Following delivery, the woman is transferred to a high-dependency area between 12 and 48 hours for close observation. Transfer to a normal labour ward is the decision of a senior staff (preferably consultants).
- Before discharge, advise about contraception. Allow her to be checked by a cardiologist and advise cardiologic follow-up after discharge.

STATION 5: MEDICAL DISORDERS WITH PREGNANCY

Obesity with pregnancy

BACKGROUND   *What obstetrician should know about obesity with pregnancy*

Risks

Risks of obesity during pregnancy include:
- Gestational diabetes
- Hypertensive disorders
- Venous thromboembolism
- Slower labour progress 4 – 10cm
- Emergency caesarean
- Postpartum haemorrhage
- Wound infection
- Birth defects
- Prematurity
- Macrosomia
- Shoulder dystocia
- Admission to neonatal care unit
- Stillbirth
- Neonatal death

Risk assessment

All maternity units should be assessed for the availability of facilities to care for obese women. Assessment includes:
- Circulation space
- Accessibility including doorway widths and thresholds
- Safe working loads of equipment (up to 250kg) and floors
- Appropriate theatre gowns
- Equipment storage
- Transportation
- Staffing levels
- Availability of specific equipment:
    - large blood pressure cuffs
    - sit-on weighing scale
    - large chairs without arms
    - large wheelchairs
    - ultrasound scan couches
    - ward and delivery beds
    - theatre trolleys
    - operating theatre tables
    - lifting and lateral transfer equipment

APPROACH   *How obstetricians should deal with obesity in Pregnancy*

I. Pre-conception care

Primary care service

- For all women during the childbearing period, advice on weight and lifestyle should be given during family planning consultations to ensure optimal body weight.
- Women are followed-up regularly by weight, body mass index and waist circumference

Women with BMI > 30?

Inform about the risks of obesity during pregnancy Support weight loss before pregnancy	Advise 5mg folic acid daily, starting at least one month before conception

II. Antenatal care

Booking visit

Measure weight, height and BMI. Report data in handheld notes and electronic patient information system.

Women with BMI > 30?

- Give information about the risk of obesity in pregnancy and how to minimize it.
- Consider thromboembolism risk and give thromboprophylaxis if indicated (repeat throughout pregnancy).
- Refer to consultant obstetrician to discuss delivery plan
- Use appropriate size cuff for BP measurement at booking visit and follow-up
- Continue folic acid till 12 weeks, give 10 mcg vitamin D during pregnancy and lactation , give 75mg aspirin if there is additional moderate risk of re-eclampsia (first pregnancy, age > 40 years, family history of pre-eclampsia, multiple pregnancy)

Further management

BMI 30 - 35	BMI > 35		BMI > 40
No additional care in the booking visit	**No additional risk of pre-eclampsia**	**Additional risk of pre-eclampsia**	Antenatal consultation & review by an obstetric anesthetist to identify potential difficulties with venous access, regional or general anaesthesia and future delivery plan
	Community monitoring every 3 weeks between 24-32 weeks and every 2 weeks till delivery	Referral to specialist input to care	**Additional risk** ← / **No additional risk of pre-eclampsia** →

24-28 weeks

Screen all women for gestational diabetes by 75g oral glucose tolerance test

Third trimester

Re-measure weight
Risk assessment for **manual handling requirements***

---

*Manual handling requirements include consideration of appropriate loads of beds and theatre tables, lateral transfer equipment, and appropriately sized thromboembolic deterrent stockings.

III. Intrapartum care

BMI 30 - 35	**BMI > 35**	**BMI > 40**
Individual risk assessment to decide the plan of birth	Advise birth in consultant-led obstetric unit	Inform duty anesthetist at delivery or intervention (midwife reports notification)

Delivery

Normal birth is encouraged (induction of labour may be associated with failure and Cesarean section which is risky) → Alert staff if weight > 120 and needs operative intervention

No obstetric contraindication to vaginal birth

Vaginal delivery

If the BMI > 40:
- Offer continuous midwifery care.
- Establish early venous access and consider early epidural analgesia
- Inform senior obstetrician and anesthetist (at least ST6). They should attend in case of operative delivery

If there is any obstetric indication

Cesarean section

- A single dose of prophylactic antibiotics is given at Cesarean section.
- A subcutaneous fat > 2 cm needs to be sutured.
- Inform senior obstetrician and anesthetist (at least ST6). They should attend Cesarean section

IV. Postpartum care

BMI 30 - 35	**BMI > 35**	**BMI > 40**

- Encourage to mobilize as early as possible.
- Encourage and support breastfeeding. Give information about benefits, initiation and maintenance of breastfeeding (less adherence to breastfeeding is recognized in obese mothers).
- Refer for future diet and life style advice

Beside other measures, give thromboprophylaxis for 7 days regardless of mode of delivery

If gestational diabetes was diagnosed

Test of glucose tolerance 6 weeks after delivery	Offer life style and weight management advice	Annual screening for type 2 diabetes and cardio-metabolic risk factors (Refer to GP)

Thrombo-prophylaxis

If ≥ 1 additional risk factors for thromboembolism, give postnatal thrombo-prophylaxis for 7 days

If ≥ 2 additional risk factors for thromboembolism, Provide compression stockings

Appendix-I   **Information given to pregnant women with BMI > 30**

- Inform about the increased risk of pre-eclampsia and gestational diabetes.
- Inform about the increased risk of fetal macrosomia and the subsequent need for obstetric care including increased level of maternal and fetal monitoring.
- Inform about potential difficulties in fetal surveillance and anomaly screening for anomalies due to poor ultrasound visualisation of the fetus.
- Inform about difficulty with intrapartum fetal monitoring, anaesthesia and caesarean section.
- Inform about the need for senior obstetric and anaesthetic involvement and an antenatal anaesthetic assessment.
- Inform about the importance of healthy eating (based on appropriately trained professional advice) and proper exercise during pregnancy .

Appendix-II | **Thromboprophylaxis for obesity during pregnancy**

A BMI ≥ 30 who also has 2 or more additional risk factors for thromboembolism should be considered for prophylactic low molecular weight heparin (LMWH) antenatally beginning early in pregnancy. They should continue prophylactic doses of LMWH until 6 weeks postpartum after postnatal risk assessment.

Weight (kg)	Dose		
	Enoxaparin	Dalteparin	Tinzaparin
91-130	60 mg daily	7500 units daily	7000 units daily
131-170	80 mg	10000 units daily	9000 units daily
>170	0.6 mg/kg/day	75 units/kg/day	75 units/kg/day

CHAPTER 6
LABOUR MANAGEMENT

STATION 6: LABOUR MANAGEMENT

Intrapartum management

| I | **PLANNING THE PLACE OF BIRTH** |

Woman should be involved in the decision of place of birth

The woman should be always informed that labour is generally very safe for the woman and the baby. The possible options should be discussed with the mother but they should be aware that available information about planning birthplace is not so evident

| Birth at home | Birth at midwife-led unit | Birth at obstetric unit |

- Birth at home provides greater chance of normal birth and less probability for intervention.
- Women should be informed about the possibility of transfer to obstetric unit and the time needed to transfer.
- There is no adequate information about the risks of home birth to the mother and the baby. However, women should be informed that if a serious event unexpectedly happens during labour at home or in a midwife-led unit, both maternal and neonatal outcomes will be worse than if they were in the obstetric unit.

- Any woman with pre-existing medical condition or a previous complicated birth is advised to deliver in an obstetric unit.
- The obstetric unit provides access to obstetricians, anaesthetists (including epidural), neonatologists and other specialists care.

| II | **INITIAL APPROACH** |

Good communication
- Knock and wait before entering her room, greet with a smile and personal welcome and introduce yourself, explain your role in care during labour.
- Establish the woman's language needs, keep calm and confident to reassure the woman that everything is going well. Ask how she is feeling.

Initial assessment
- Listen to the woman and ask her about vaginal loss and contractions
- Review clinical records
- General examination: check vital signs and urinalysis
- Abdominal examination: observe contractions, fetal heart rate (FHR) and palpate abdomen
- Vaginal examination is offered.

If the woman is not in labour, reassure, offer individualised support and encourage her to return home

End of initial approach
- If the woman has a written birth plan, read and discuss it with her.
- Discuss options of coping with pain with her and discuss all potential procedures and observations to take her permission.
- Encourage the woman to adapt her individual needs. Tell the woman and her partner how to call for help.
- When leaving the room, let her know when to return.

III   INTRAPARTUM MANAGEMENT*

First stage of labour

Once the onset of labour is diagnosed, use a partogram (with a 4-hour action line) to follow-up labour progress
Consider the woman's emotional and psychological needs

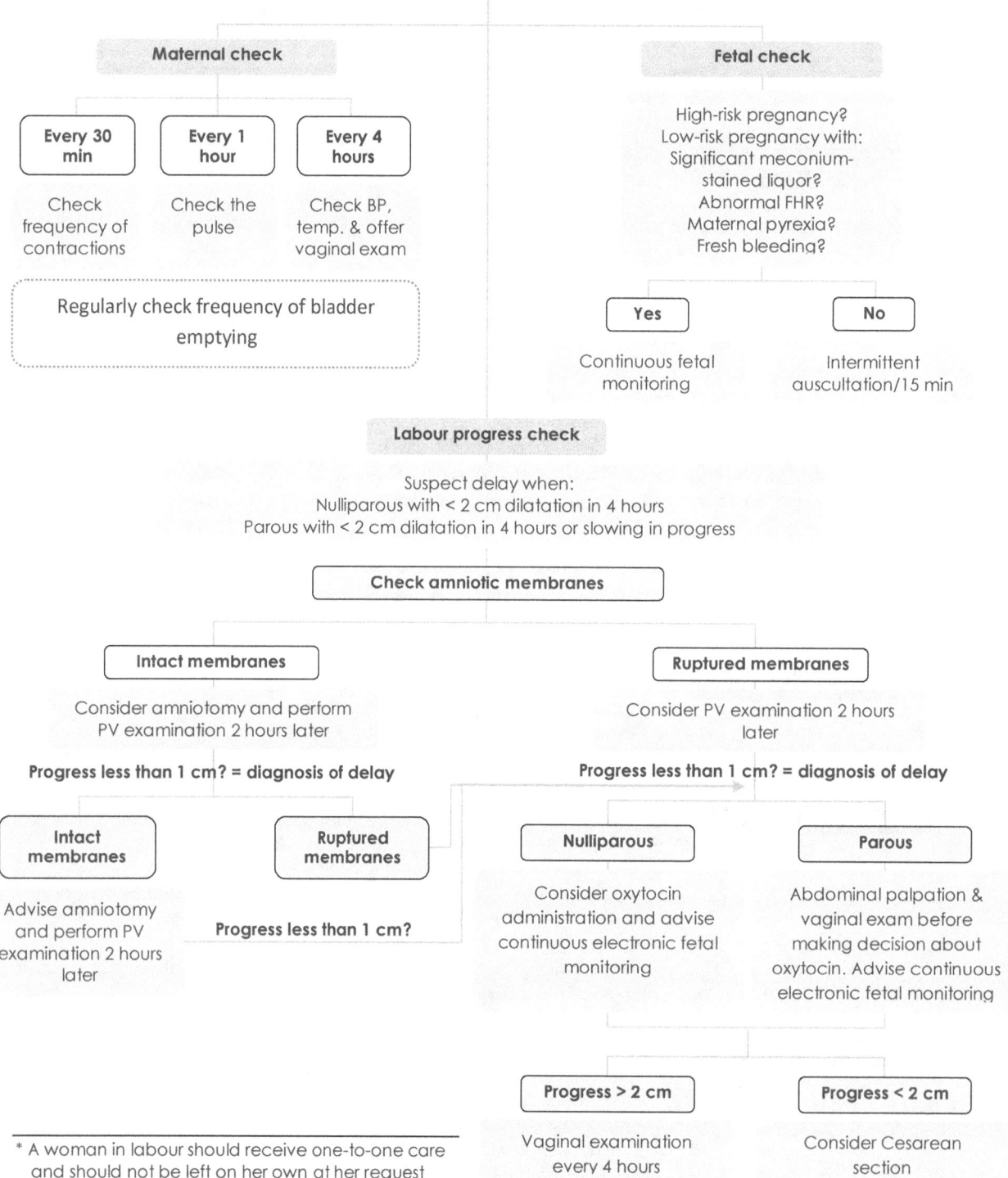

Maternal check

Every 30 min	Every 1 hour	Every 4 hours
Check frequency of contractions	Check the pulse	Check BP, temp. & offer vaginal exam

Regularly check frequency of bladder emptying

Fetal check

High-risk pregnancy?
Low-risk pregnancy with:
Significant meconium-stained liquor?
Abnormal FHR?
Maternal pyrexia?
Fresh bleeding?

Yes	No
Continuous fetal monitoring	Intermittent auscultation/15 min

Labour progress check

Suspect delay when:
Nulliparous with < 2 cm dilatation in 4 hours
Parous with < 2 cm dilatation in 4 hours or slowing in progress

Check amniotic membranes

Intact membranes

Consider amniotomy and perform PV examination 2 hours later

Progress less than 1 cm? = diagnosis of delay

Intact membranes

Advise amniotomy and perform PV examination 2 hours later

Ruptured membranes

Progress less than 1 cm?

Ruptured membranes

Consider PV examination 2 hours later

Progress less than 1 cm? = diagnosis of delay

Nulliparous

Consider oxytocin administration and advise continuous electronic fetal monitoring

Parous

Abdominal palpation & vaginal exam before making decision about oxytocin. Advise continuous electronic fetal monitoring

Progress > 2 cm

Vaginal examination every 4 hours

Progress < 2 cm

Consider Cesarean section

* A woman in labour should receive one-to-one care and should not be left on her own at her request and for short periods only.

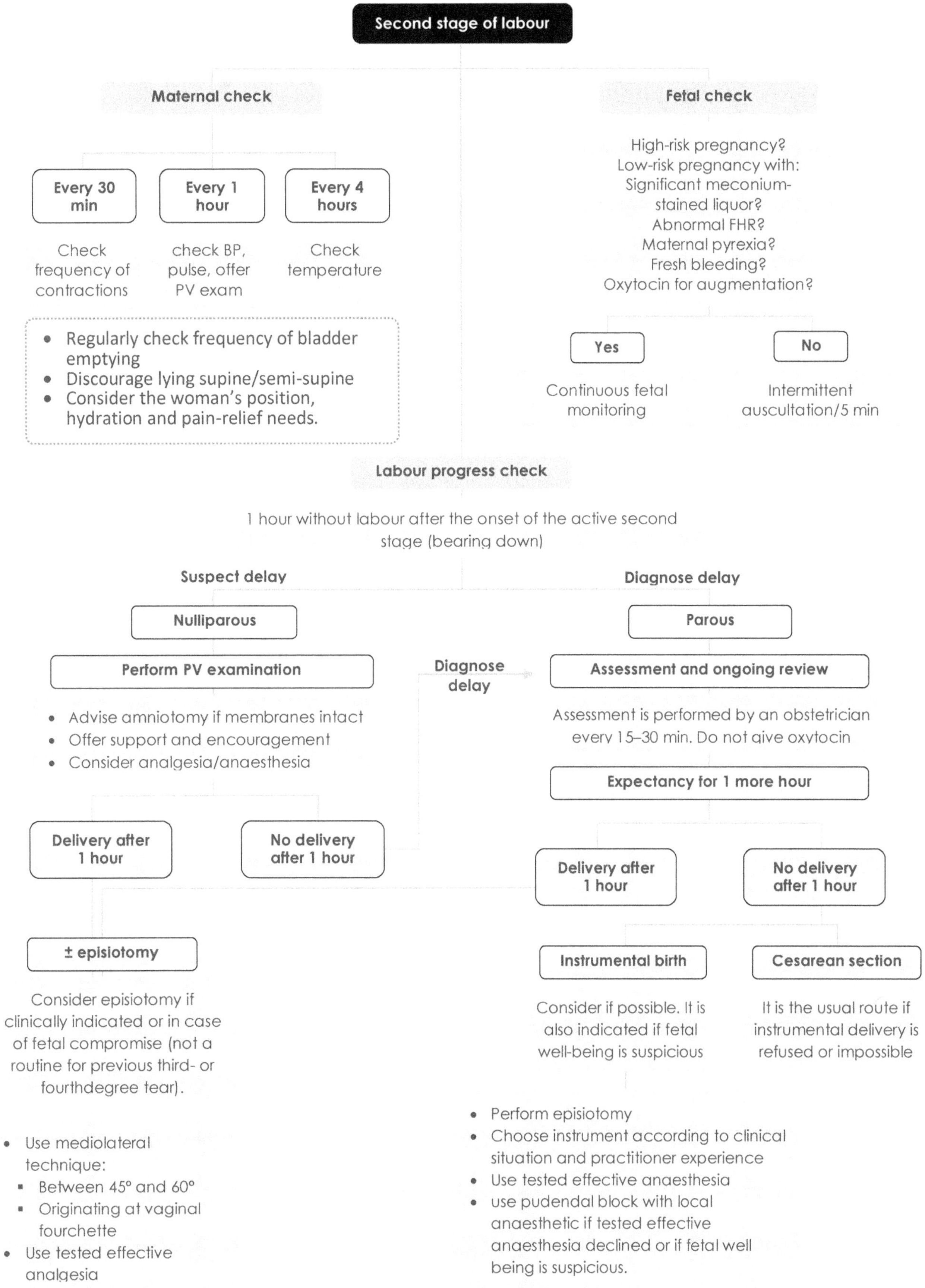

Second stage of labour

Maternal check

Every 30 min	Every 1 hour	Every 4 hours
Check frequency of contractions	check BP, pulse, offer PV exam	Check temperature

- Regularly check frequency of bladder emptying
- Discourage lying supine/semi-supine
- Consider the woman's position, hydration and pain-relief needs.

Fetal check

High-risk pregnancy?
Low-risk pregnancy with:
Significant meconium-stained liquor?
Abnormal FHR?
Maternal pyrexia?
Fresh bleeding?
Oxytocin for augmentation?

Yes	No
Continuous fetal monitoring	Intermittent auscultation/5 min

Labour progress check

1 hour without labour after the onset of the active second stage (bearing down)

Suspect delay

Nulliparous

Perform PV examination

- Advise amniotomy if membranes intact
- Offer support and encouragement
- Consider analgesia/anaesthesia

Delivery after 1 hour	No delivery after 1 hour

± episiotomy

Consider episiotomy if clinically indicated or in case of fetal compromise (not a routine for previous third- or fourthdegree tear).

- Use mediolateral technique:
  ▪ Between 45° and 60°
  ▪ Originating at vaginal fourchette
- Use tested effective analgesia

Diagnose delay →

Diagnose delay

Parous

Assessment and ongoing review

Assessment is performed by an obstetrician every 15–30 min. Do not give oxytocin

Expectancy for 1 more hour

Delivery after 1 hour	No delivery after 1 hour

Instrumental birth	Cesarean section
Consider if possible. It is also indicated if fetal well-being is suspicious	It is the usual route if instrumental delivery is refused or impossible

- Perform episiotomy
- Choose instrument according to clinical situation and practitioner experience
- Use tested effective anaesthesia
- use pudendal block with local anaesthetic if tested effective anaesthesia declined or if fetal well being is suspicious.

Third stage of labour

Check

Check maternal general condition and vaginal loss

Placental delivery

Active management

It is the usual route because it reduces risk of haemorrhage and shortens third stage

- Oxytocin (10 IU IM).
- Early cord clamping/cutting
- Controlled cord traction

No placenta delivery for 30 minutes

Physiologic management

It is the route only if requested by low-risk woman.

- No oxytocin (just maternal effort)
- No early cord clamping
- Do not pull cord or palpate uterus

No placenta delivery for 1 hour

Convert to active management

Give Oxytocin (10 IU IM) and apply Controlled cord traction

No placenta delivery

Obtain IV access and give oxytocin

Inject 20 IU in 20 ml of saline into the umbilical vein (no IV oxytocin infusion) with proximal cord clamping

No placenta delivery for 30 minutes

Assessment

Use analgesia or anaesthesia for assessment. Stop assessment if there is inadequate pain relief and address that.

Manual removal

Manual removal of the placenta under effective regional or general anaesthesia

Postpartum care

Maternal care

Check the placenta, the cord and membranes for anomalies or residual intrauterine parts

Ask how she feels

General assessment

Check vital signs, emotional and psychological condition

Local assessment

Check uterine contractions, lochia, and bladder voiding.

Perineal check

Perform systematic assessment of any perineal trauma including a rectal examination. Consider:

- Explaining assessment to the woman
- Confirming that analgesia is effective.
- Lithotomy, if required, only for assessment and repair

Document extent and findings

First degree	Suture skin if not well opposed using continuous subcuticular technique
Second degree	Suture vaginal wall & muscle with continuous non-locked sutures, skin as above
Third degree	Seek obstetrician advice (transfer to obstetric unit if appropriate)
Fourth degree	Seek obstetrician advice (transfer to obstetric unit if appropriate)

Consider rectal NSAIDs for analgesia following perineal repair

Newborn care

Keep the baby worm and check the APGAR score at 1 and 5 minutes to assess the need for resuscitation

Resuscitation*

- Start basic resuscitation of newborn babies with air.
- Use oxygen for babies who do not respond.

Within 1 hour

- Encourage skin-to-skin contact as soon as possible and do not separate the mother and the baby in the first hour.
- Initiate breast-feeding

After 1 hour

Record baby's head circumference, body temperature and weight

* Attend a neonatal resuscitation course at least once a year

Fact Box: amniotomy and oxytocin

- **Amniotomy:**
  Before performing amniotomy, explain the procedure and its purposes to the woman. The main advantages of amniotomy are:
    - Shortening of labour (by about an hour)
    - Making contractions stronger and more painful
- **Oxytocin:**
  Before giving oxytocin, explain the purposes and withdraws to the woman. This includes:
    - Oxytocin will hasten birth but does not influence mode of birth.
    - It increases frequency and strength of contractions.
    - Continuous EFM will be indicated.
  Offer epidural anaesthesia before starting oxytocin, Oxytocin increments every 30 min until 4–5 contractions in 10 minutes are obtained.

Fact Box: Indications of transfer to an obstetric unit

Indications of transfer to an obstetric unit includes:
- *Indications for electronic fetal monitoring (EFM):* see later.
- *Fetal heartbeat:* is uncertain.
- *Malpresentations:* diagnosed for the first time at the onset of labour.
- *Obstetric emergency:* antepartum haemorrhage, cord presentation and prolapse, postpartum haemorrhage, maternal collapse or advanced neonatal resuscitation
- *Raised blood pressure:* raised diastolic blood pressure (over 90 mmHg) or systolic blood pressure (over 140 mmHg) on two consecutive measurements taken 30 minutes apart.
- *Complications after birth:* Retained placenta, third- or fourth-degree tear or other perineal trauma that indicate suturing

Appendix - I   **Management of pain during labour**

Encouragement and support

Encourage women to ask for analgesia at any time during labour. Consider your attitude and the woman's choice for pain control.

Labouring in water	Breathing/relaxation techniques, massage, music	Acupuncture, acupressure and hypnosis	Transcutaneous electrical nerve stimulation
Labouring in water is encouraged to reduce pain during labour	These options should be always supported to reduce pain throughout labour	These methods are not be provided. However, do not prevent women if they want to use them	This should not be offered to women who are already in labour

Discuss analgesic options

Inhalation analgesia and opioids

Consider Entonox and opioids (pethidine or diamorphine) for analgesia. However, you should explain to the mother that these options achieve limited pain relief.

Entonox

Entonox may cause nausea and light-headedness

Opioids

Opioids may cause:
- **Maternal:** drowsiness, nausea and vomiting in the mother and may interfere with breastfeeding.
- **Neonatal:** may cause short-term respiratory depression and drowsiness for days. Provide antiemetic. Advise no birthing pool or bath within 2 hours or if drowsy.

After each bolus, measure BP every 5 min for 15 min

After each bolus, provide continuous EFM for 30 minutes

After 30 min, call anaesthetist if pain persists

Every hour, check level of sensory block

In the 2nd stage, no routine oxytocin. Delay pushing for 1 hr

In the 3rd stage, continue epidural until any perineal repair

Epidural anesthesia

Counseling

Inform women that:
- It is more effective than opioids
- It is only available in obstetric units
- It prolongs the second (not first) stage of labour and increases the risk of instrumental birth (not CS).
- There is no long-term backache
- It indicates more intensive monitoring and IV access
- If a large amount of opioid is used, it may cause short-term respiratory problems and drowsiness in the baby.

Preparation

Obtain IV access. Do not give preloading or maintenance fluid infusion as a routine

Achievement

- Use epidural or combined spinal–epidural analgesia. Use combined spinal/epidural analgesia(bupivacaine and fentanyl) for rapid relief
- Use low-concentration anaesthetic and opioid to initiate and maintain epidural
- Do not use high concentrations of local anaesthetics routinely
- 2nd stage should be completed in 4 hours

Encourage any comfortable upright

STATION 6: LABOUR MANAGEMENT

Intrapartum fetal assessment

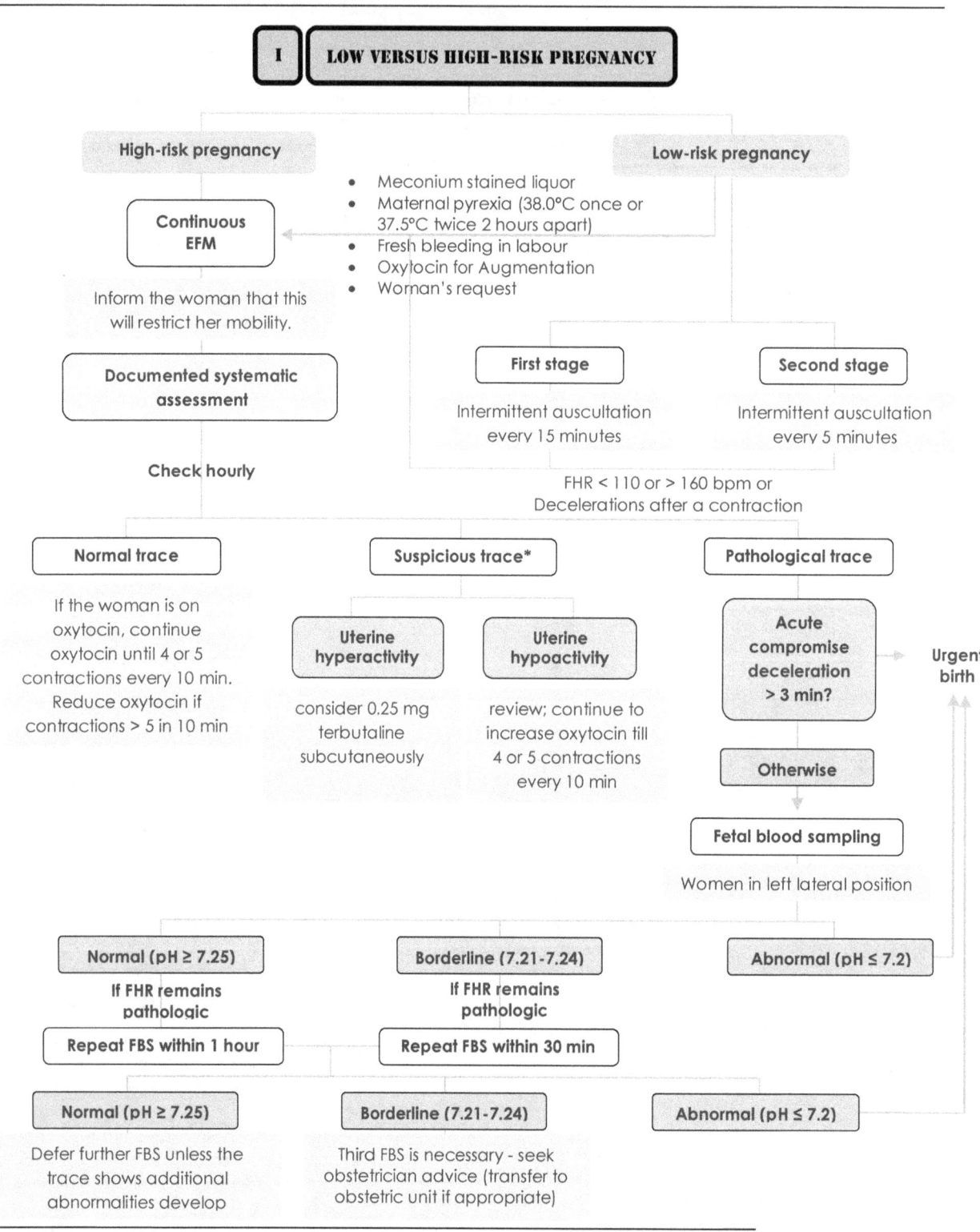

| I | LOW VERSUS HIGH-RISK PREGNANCY |

High-risk pregnancy

Low-risk pregnancy

- Meconium stained liquor
- Maternal pyrexia (38.0°C once or 37.5°C twice 2 hours apart)
- Fresh bleeding in labour
- Oxytocin for Augmentation
- Woman's request

Continuous EFM

Inform the woman that this will restrict her mobility.

Documented systematic assessment

Check hourly

First stage

Intermittent auscultation every 15 minutes

Second stage

Intermittent auscultation every 5 minutes

FHR < 110 or > 160 bpm or Decelerations after a contraction

Normal trace

If the woman is on oxytocin, continue oxytocin until 4 or 5 contractions every 10 min. Reduce oxytocin if contractions > 5 in 10 min

Suspicious trace*

Uterine hyperactivity

consider 0.25 mg terbutaline subcutaneously

Uterine hypoactivity

review; continue to increase oxytocin till 4 or 5 contractions every 10 min

Pathological trace

Acute compromise deceleration > 3 min?

Urgent birth

Otherwise

Fetal blood sampling

Women in left lateral position

Normal (pH ≥ 7.25)

If FHR remains pathologic

Repeat FBS within 1 hour

Borderline (7.21-7.24)

If FHR remains pathologic

Repeat FBS within 30 min

Abnormal (pH ≤ 7.2)

Normal (pH ≥ 7.25)

Defer further FBS unless the trace shows additional abnormalities develop

Borderline (7.21-7.24)

Third FBS is necessary - seek obstetrician advice (transfer to obstetric unit if appropriate)

Abnormal (pH ≤ 7.2)

* If there is suspicion of fetal death: confirm fetal viability by real time ultrasound

Parameters of electronic FHR monitoring assessment

Reassuring features

- Baseline rate = 110-160 bpm
- Variability ≥ 5 bpm
- Accelerations are present
- Decelerations are absent

Non-reassuring features

- Baseline rate = 100-109 bpm or 161-180 bpm
- Variability < 5 bpm for 40-90 minutes
- Accelerations are absent*
- Decelerations either:
  - Typical variable decelerations with > 50% of contractions, for > 90 min
  - Single prolonged deceleration for up to 3 min

Abnormal features

- Baseline rate < 100 bpm or >180 bpm. Sinusoidal pattern > 10 minutes
- Variability < 5 bpm for 90 minutes
- Accelerations are absent*
- Decelerations either:
  - Atypical variable decelerations with > 50% of contractions, for > 30 min
  - Late decelerations with > 50% of contractions for > 30 min
  - Single prolonged deceleration for > 3 min

| All features of the trace are reassuring | One non-reassuring feature | 2 or more non-reassuring features | One or more abnormal features |

| **Normal trace** | **Suspicious trace** | | **Pathological trace** |

---

* Absence of accelerations alone is of uncertain significance if the other features of the trace are normal

| II | **MECONIUM-STAINED LIQUOR** |

Light meconium-stained liquor

Liquor with light greenish discoloration but no thick meconium revealed

Consider continuous EFM

Consider continuous EFM based on risk assessment*

Management according to trace features (see before)

Newborn care

Check for neonatal well-being at 1 and 2 hours if the baby is in a good condition. Check the following:
- General wellbeing
- Heart rate and respiration and temperature
- Chest movements and nasal flare
- Skin colour and capillary refill
- Feeding
- Muscle tone

Any concern develops at any time?

Review by a neonatologist

Significant meconium-stained liquor

Dark green or black thick or tenacious liquor or meconium lumps in liquor **

Advise continuous EFM

Confirm FBS availability during labour and advanced neonatal life support at birth

Birth

- Avoid nasopharynx and oropharynx suction before delivery of the shoulders and trunk
- Perform upper airway suction if there is thick meconium in oropharynx.

Good general conditions

Check at 1 hour, 2 hours then 2-hourly (until 12 hours). Check:
- General wellbeing
- Heart rate and respiration and temperature
- Chest movements and nasal flare
- Skin colour and capillary refill
- Feeding
- Muscle tone

Depressed vital signs

Suction under direct vision using laryngoscopy

This is performed by a healthcare professional in advanced neonatal life support

---

* This includes consideration of stage of labour, volume of liquor, parity, FHR and transfer pathway
** seek obstetrician advice (transfer to obstetric unit)

STATION 6: LABOUR MANAGEMENT

Shoulder dystocia

BACKGROUND   *What obstetrician should know basically about shoulder dystocia*

Definitions

It is a complication to vaginal cephalic delivery, which requires specific obstetric manoeuvres to deliver the fetus after delivery of the fetus when gentle traction has failed to deliver the shoulders of the fetus.

Risk factors

Antepartum risks

- Diabetes mellitus
- Maternal body mass index > 30kg/m²
- Previous shoulder dystocia
- Macrosomia (more than 4.5kg)

Intrapartum risks

- Induction of labour
- Oxytocin augmentation
- Assisted vaginal delivery
- Prolonged first stage of labour
- Secondary arrest
- Prolonged second stage of labour

Complications

Maternal complications

- Postpartum haemorrhage (11%)
- Third and fourth-degree perineal tears (3.8%)

Maternal complications are not related to the number and nature of manoeuvres that are made to deliver the fetus.

Fetal complications

- Brachial plexus injury (BPI) in 2.3% to 16%

BPI is the most common cause in litigation in cases of shoulder dystocia. The following facts about shoulder dystocia should be well known:

- Most cases of BPI resolve without permanent disability. Only < 10% of cases may suffer permanent problems. Large infants are more susceptible.
- BPI is not always associated with malpractice. About 46% of cases may be associated with substandard care. Maternal propulsive force may contribute to this complication in some cases.
- BPIs are not always associated with shoulder dystocia. About 4-12 % of injuries were reported after uncomplicated caesarean section.
- As a medico-legal issue, the shoulder that was affected at the time of birth should be reported clearly because BPIs in the posterior shoulder are unlikely to be caused by a healthcare professional.

APPROACH   *How obstetricians should deal with shoulder dystocia*

First   **Prevention of shoulder dystocia**

Prediction

Prophylactic intervention

General risk assessment

Identification of pre-existing risk factors prior to labour

Insufficient prediction

❶ They predict only 16% of cases
❷ Most fetuses weighing > 4.5 Kg do not develop shoulder dystocia
❸ 48% cases of shoulder dystocia develop in fetuses < 4 kg.

The single most important risk factor is maternal diabetes (2-4 fold increase in risk)

Selected risk model

A combination of certain risk factors as a scoring sheet

Better prediction?

A combination of maternal height, weight, gestational age, parity and birth weight are used. They may predict 50.7% of cases of shoulder dystocia (from one retrospective study)

ALWAYS REMEMBER: there is a 10% potential error in fetal weight estimation by ultrasound*

Consider prophylactic procedure under certain circumstances

Consider induction of labour

There is no rule of prophylactic McRoberts' manoeuvre before head delivery to prevents shoulder dystocia

Induction of labour should be considered in **diabetic** mothers with normally grown fetuses after 38 weeks of gestations. This is NOT applied to non-diabetic women with suspected macrosomia

?

Consider Cesarean section

Elective Cesarean section should be considered in **diabetic** mothers with fetuses > 4.5 Kg. It may also be recommended in non-diabetic women with fetal weight > 5 kg (consider ultrasound errors)

Previous shoulder dystocia?

There is no definite recommendation about the route of delivery in these cases. Management depends on the severity of previous neonatal or maternal injury, the current predicted fetal size and finally on maternal counseling. The recurrent risk of shoulder dystocia is 10 times the general population (1-25%)

---

*This risk model depends on actual rather than estimated fetal weight

Second Management of shoulder dystocia

Birth attendants

Birth attendants should be aware how to diagnose shoulder dystocia and how to perform the maneuvers that facilitate fetal delivery

> Difficulty with delivery of the face and chin?

> The head remaining tightly applied to the vulva or even retracting (turtle-neck sign)?

> Failure of restitution of the fetal head?

> Failure of the shoulders to descend?

Suspect shoulder dystocia

Apply routine axial traction (in line with fetal spine) and not lateral traction to avoid nerve avulsion

Failed?

Diagnose shoulder dystocia

Discourage maternal pushing
Avoid fundal pressure
Encourage the woman to lie flat, move the buttocks to the table edge

> Call for help

Call a midwife coordinator - additional midwife - experienced obstetrician - obstetric anaesthetist - neonatal team

> McRoberts' manoeuvre
> +
> Supra-pubic pressure

Apply routine axial traction

Failed?

Management according to circumstances and experience (same efficiency)

> Deliver the posterior arm

> Internal rotation procedures

The fetal wrist is grasped and withdrawn gently in a straight line (2-12% risk of humeral fracture)

Consider Episiotomy only if a space is needed for maneuvers

Pressing the posterior (or anterior) aspects of the posterior shoulder into the oblique diameter of the pelvis

Involve consultant obstetrician and anesthetist

Failed?

> All fours position
> OR
> Repeat the scheme again

Failed?

> Third line management including cleidotomy, symphysiotomy or Zavanelli

❶ **The McRoberts' manoeuvre**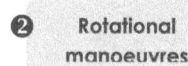

- **The manoeuvre:**

  This manoeuvre involves flexion and abduction of the maternal hips to place the thighs on the abdomen.

- **Mechanism (rationale):**

  - This manoeuvre straightens the lumbosacral angle.
  - It also rotates the maternal pelvis upwards.
  - It also increases the anterior-posterior diameter of the pelvis.

- **Steps:**

  - The woman is placed flat.
  - The woman's legs are removed from the supports (if any).
  - The woman's legs are hyperflexed with the aid of 2 assistants on each side.
  - Routine axial traction is then applied to the fetal head to assess release of the shoulders from the maternal pelvis.

- **Success rate:**

  It reaches up to 90%.

- **Complications:**

  It has a low rate of complications because it does not involve internal manoeuvres.

Suprapubic pressure

- **The manoeuvre:**

  Suprapubic pressure may be applied along with the McRoberts' manoeuvre to increase the chance of success.

- **Mechanism (rationale):**

  - This manoeuvre minimizes the descending fetal bisacromial diameter through the pelvis (pushing the anterior shoulder towards the pelvis).
  - It also rotates the anterior shoulder into the oblique pelvic diameter.

- **Steps:**

  - An assistant applies pressure just above the maternal symphysis pubis from the side of the fetal back. The direction of pressure is downward and lateral.
  - The pressure may be continuous or intermittent (rocking). No method is superior to the other.

❷ **Rotational manoeuvres**

- **The manoeuvre: (Woods and Rubin)**

  Gaining access through the vagina is made to press on the posterior shoulder (either on the anterior or posterior aspect).

- **Mechanism:**

  - This manoeuvre brings the shoulders into the wider oblique diameter.
  - If the posterior aspect of the posterior shoulder is pressed, this also adducts the shoulders and reduces the shoulder diameter.

- **Steps:**

  - Pressure is best applied on the posterior aspect of the posterior shoulder.
  - If this fails, an attempt to apply pressure on the posterior aspect of the anterior shoulder should be made.

❸ Posterior arm delivery

- **The manoeuvre:**
  Gaining access through the vagina is made to bring the posterior arm through the pelvis into the vagina.
- **Mechanism:**
  The manoeuvre brings the width of the arm below the pelvic inlet and thus reduces the diameter of the fetal shoulders.
- **Steps:**
  - The hand of the operator is inserted through the vagina and the fetal wrist is grasped.
  - The posterior arm is gently withdrawn following a straight line.
- **Complications:**
  - Humeral fractures (2% - 12%). However, this is controversial. It may be attributed to the procedure or to the condition itself.
  - Generally, it was reported that the incidence of both BPI and humeral fractures is higher than in those who were managed by rotational methods.

Episiotomy

- There is no rule of episiotomy to facilitate shoulder delivery because it involves soft tissues rather than pelvic bone, which prevents shoulder descent. Accordingly, episiotomy does not decrease the incidence of shoulder dystocia or its complications including BPI.
- Episiotomy is only indicated if it is going to help the operator to perform internal procedures by allowing more space for these manoeuvres.

❹ All fours position

The All fours position is suitable in certain circumstances. If the woman is slim, mobile and without epidural anaesthesia specially with a single attending midwife, this position may be attended. Otherwise, internal manoeuvres are more appropriate.

❺ Third line procedures

① **Cleidotomy:** surgically induced clavicle fracture or bending of the clavicle with a finger).

② **Symphysiotomy:** dividing the anterior fibres of symphyseal ligament to widen the pelvis.

This procedure is helpful. However, it may cause serious maternal morbidity. Furthermore, the neonatal outcome is generally poor.

③ **Zavanelli manoeuvre (rare):** pushing the head through the vagina then caesarean section to deliver the fetus.

- *Advantages:*
  This procedure is best resorted to bilateral shoulder dystocia (one shoulder above the symphysis pubis and the other above the sacral promontory).
- *Disadvantages:*
  The procedure is difficult and time consuming; the risk of hypoxic ischaemic injury is low within 5 minutes but becomes significant thereafter.

Third   **Postpartum management**

Maternal evaluation

Fetal evaluation

The following should be carefully checked in all women after delivery:

- Postpartum haemorrhage
- 3rd and 4th degree perineal tears
- Other injuries including vaginal and cervical tears
- Organ rupture including bladder rupture and uterine rupture
- Bony pelvis injuries including symphyseal separation and sacroiliac joint dislocation
- Neurological deficits i.e. lateral femoral cutaneous neuropathy

The newborn should be checked for the following:

- BPI
- Other fetal injuries e.g. humeral and clavicle fractures
- Pneumothoraces
- Hypoxic brain damage (particularly after 5 minutes).

Documentation

Adequate and comprehensive documentation of manoeuvres should be made. The whole birth event should be explained carefully to the parents

Acknowledgement:

The Royal College of Obstetricians and Gynaecologists (RCOG) green-top and National Institute for Health and Care Excellence (NICE) were the main source of preparation of this work. Thank you for supplying these free sources for us. Our target is to help young physicians and MRCOG exam candidates to digest the prcinciples of good practice after reading the original sources available in RCOG and NICE guidelines

Additional references:

1- Harper PS. Practical Genetic Counseling. 4th edition.Woburn: Butterworth-Heinemann, 1993.

2- Main DN, Mennuti MT. Neural tube defects: issues in prenatal diagnosis and counseling. Obstet Gynecol 1986;67:1-15.

3- Loeken M: Current perspectives on the causes of neural tube defects resulting from diabetic pregnancy. Am J Med Genet Part C (Semin Med Genet) 135C:77, 2005.

4- Zhao Z, Reece EA: Experimental mechanisms of diabetic embryopathy and strategies for developing therapeutic interventions. J Soc Gynecol Invest 12:449, 2005.

5- Canadian Task Force on the Periodic Health Examination. Periodic Health Examination, 1994 update: 3. Primary and secondary prevention of neural tube defects. Can Med Assoc J 1994;151:159-66.

6- Feichtbam LB, Cunningham G,Waller DK, Lustig LS,Tompkinson DG, Hook EB. Fetal karyotyping for chromosome abnormalities after an unexplained elevated maternal serum alpha-fetoprotein screening. Obstet Gynecol 1995;986:248-54.

7- Thiagarajah S, Stroud CB, Babelidis F, Schnorr JA, Schnatterly PT, Ferguson JE. Elevated maternal serum alpha-fetoprotein levels: what is the risk of fetal aneuploidy? Am J Obstet Gynecol 1995;713:388-9.

8- Royal College of Obstetricians and Gynaecologists. Amniocentesis and Chorionic Villus Sampling. London:RCOG; June 2010.

9- Baird PA, Sadovnick AD: Survival in infants with anencephaly. Clin Pediatr 23: 268, 1984.

10- Royal College of Obstetricians and Gynaecologists. Termination of Pregnancy for Fetal Abnormality in England, Scotland and Wales. London:RCOG; May 1010.

11- Anteby EY, Yagel S: Route of delivery of fetuses with structural anomalies. Eur J Obstet Gynecol Reprod Biol 2003; 106; 5-9.

12- ACOG Practice Bulletin. Screening for fetal chromosomal abnormalities. Obstet Gynecol. 109(1), Jan 2007.

13- Tolmie J. Down syndrome and other autosomal trisomies. In: Rimoin DL, Connor JM, Pyeritz RE, Korf BR. Emery and Rimoin's Principles and Practice of Medical Genetics. 4th edition. 2002:1129-1183.

14- Update on carrier screening for cystic fibrosis. Committee Opinion No. 486. American College of Obstetricians and Gynecologists. Obstet Gynecol 2011 ;117:1028-31.

15- J Livingstone, R A Axton, A Gilfillan, et al. Antenatal screening for cystic fibrosis: a trial of the couple model. BMJ 1994;308:1459.

16- Hong Kong College of Obstetricians and Gynaecologists guidelines. Guidelines of Antenatal Thalassaemia Screening. Oct. 2003.

17- Wenstrom KD, Weiner CP, Williamson RA, et al: Prenatal diagnosis of fetal hyperthyroidism using funipuncture. Obstet Gynecol 76:513, 1990.

18- New MI, Nimkarn S: 21-hydroxylase-deficient urogenital adrenal hyperplasia. Gene Review www.genetests.org Updated 7 September 2007.

19- Simpson JL: Fetal arrhythmias. Ultrasound Obstet Gynecol 27:599, 2006.

20- O'Brien B, Bianchi DW: Fetal therapy for single gene disorders. Clin Obstet Gynecol 48:885, 2005.

21- Irons MB, Nores J, Stewart TL, et al: Antenatal therapy of Smith-Lemli-Opitz syndrome. Fetal Diagn Ther 14:133, 1999.

22- de Koning TJ, Klomp LW, van Oppen AC, et al: Prenatal and early postnatal treatment in 3-phosphoglycerate-dehydrogenase deficiency. Lancet 364:2221, 2004.

23- Tiblad E, Westgren M: Fetal stem-cell transplantation. Best Pract Res Clin Obstet Gynaecol 22:189, 2008.